PHLEBOTOMY TECHNIQUES

A Laboratory Workbook

Susan Phelan, MHS, MT(ASCP)

This project was supported in part by a grant from Becton Dickinson VACUTAINER Systems, Rutherford, New Jersey. VACUTAINER, HEMOGARD, Unopette, Safety Flow Lancet, Bactec and SST are trademarks of Becton Dickinson and Company.

BECTON
DICKINSON

PHLEBOTOMY TECHNIQUES

A Laboratory Workbook

Susan Phelan, MHS, MT(ASCP)
Coordinator, Phlebotomy Program
Moraine Valley Community College

American Society of Clinical Pathologists

Chicago

Acquisition & Development: Joshua Weikersheimer
Editor: Karen D. Johnson
Designer: Michael Methe
Medical Illustrator: Andrea Meenahan
Marketing Manager: Denise St. John

Notice: Trade names and equipment and supplies described herein are included as suggestions only. In no way does their inclusion constitute an endorsement or preference by the American Society of Clinical Pathologists. The ASCP did not test the equipment, supplies, or procedures and, therefore, urges all readers to read and follow all manufacturer's instructions and package insert warnings concerning the proper and safe use of all products.

Library of Congress Cataloging in Publication Data

Phelan, Susan E., 1954–
Phlebotomy techniques: a laboratory workbook/
Susan Phelan.
p. cm.
Includes bibliographical references.
ISBN 0-89189-343-1
1. Phlebotomy—Laboratory manuals. I. Title.
[DNLM: 1. Bloodletting—methods—programmed instruction. WB 25 P538p]
RB45.15.P47 1992
616.07'561—dc20
DNLM/DLC
for Library of Congress 92-10957
CIP

Printed in the United States of America.
97 96 95 94 93 5 4 3 2 1

Dedication

To my husband, Robert (Sonny); our children, Robert, Meghann, and Christopher; and my parents, Selma and the late William Evers

Contents

Acknowledgments

The motivation for this book was to develop a tool designed to teach phlebotomy techniques for use in the classroom setting. The contents of this book have evolved over a period of 6 years and correspond to the development of the Moraine Valley Community College Phlebotomy Program. Several people were and continue to be instrumental in the ongoing development of this program.

First and foremost, I would like to acknowledge my mentors at Moraine Valley Community College: Suzanne Hammersberg, EdD, MT(ASCP), Dean of Public Service, Allied Health and Nursing, and Raymond Lehner, Department Chairperson, Allied Health. Dr. Hammersberg and Mr. Lehner have been most helpful and encouraging in the development of the program. In addition, they have provided insight and wise direction in applying the expertise gained in phlebotomy education at Moraine Valley Community College to the field of phlebotomy.

I would also like to acknowledge the clinical coordinators associated with the Moraine Valley Community College Phlebotomy Program. I am privileged to work with an esteemed group of knowledgeable and dedicated professionals. The clinical coordinators are wonderful about providing information to keep the phlebotomy program's curriculum current. The clinical coordinators and the facility with which they are associated are as follows: Mark Schoener and Arlene Widner, Central Medical Laboratories; Betty O'Neal and Ruby Payton, Christ Hospital and Medical Center; Sharla Parker, Community Hospital; Rasa Aleksiunas and Donna Parker, Holy Cross Hospital; Sandy Sabin and Sandy Veronese, Kendon Medical Laboratories; Audrey Blondell and Colette Schrank, Little Company of Mary Hospital; Joellyn Farina and Linda Scott, Loyola University; Mary Hejmanowski, Alex McGuinn, and Nancy Nowasczyk, Palos Community Hospital; Elyce Perry, St. Francis Hospital; Denise Demattie, Silver Cross Hospital; and Laura Savant, South Suburban Hospital.

I have been privileged to share teaching responsibilities with several dedicated and motivated instructors. I would like to acknowledge them for their impact on phlebotomy education at Moraine Valley Community College: Marion Kelly,

MS, MT(ASCP), Bertha Malone, MHS, MT(ASCP), Raymond Olesinski, MHPE, MT(ASCP)PBT,SH, CLS(NCA), and Colette Schrank, MS, MT(ASCP).

I would also like to express my appreciation to the persons directly involved with the development of *Phlebotomy Techniques: A Laboratory Workbook*. The staff at ASCP Press has provided invaluable advice and assistance in the development of this project. It is a rare privilege to work with such a talented group of people. I would specifically like to acknowledge Karen Johnson, Andrea Meenahan, Michael Methe, Denise St. John, and Joshua Weikersheimer for their many notable contributions to this project.

I would like to acknowledge Robert Braun, MT(ASCP)SBB, from Christ Hospital and Medical Center and Alex McGuinn, MT(ASCP), from Palos Community Hospital. Mr. Braun was instrumental in the development of the donor lab, and Ms. McGuinn graciously arranged for a photography session at Palos Community Hospital. Finally, I would like to gratefully acknowledge Raymond Olesinski, MHPE, MT(ASCP)PBT,SH, CLS(NCA), of the University of Kentucky, Center for Rural Health, for contributing Appendix 2, "Blood Tests and Collection Requirements," and for graciously agreeing to act as reviewer of this document before it went to press.

Introduction

This workbook is designed to provide the phlebotomy student with instruction in phlebotomy techniques, and it will address skills in psychomotor, affective, and didactic domains.

The fundamental purpose of the workbook is to provide instruction in the psychomotor domain as it relates to the practice of phlebotomy. Upon completion of the workbook, the student will possess an orientation to basic phlebotomy procedures, including skin puncture, venipuncture, arterial puncture, and bleeding times. The learner will have mastered, through repetition, certain skills considered standard to the practice of phlebotomy.

The affective domain is incorporated into the workbook through value clarification techniques and a series of role-playing exercises. Values clarification exercises are designed to assist the student in the development and internalization of a personal concept of professionalism.

Phlebotomists enjoy a unique position in laboratory medicine. Through constant patient interaction and contact, they see firsthand the benefits of laboratory medicine to the patient. In addition, phlebotomists have an important public relations role. The phlebotomist is the patient's "window" to the laboratory. The patient's perception of the quality of laboratory services and, in fact, the quality of overall care, will be determined, at least in part, on the patient's perception of the phlebotomist.

The phlebotomist routinely interacts with many different people. It is critical that students learn the interpersonal skills necessary to interact with patients and other health care workers in a professional manner. Role-playing exercises introduce the development of the interpersonal skills that the student will need when working as a phlebotomist and are incorporated into the procedures in each laboratory exercise. In this manner, students will develop confidence in their communication skills through repetition and practice. In addition, situations requiring advanced communication skills will be presented. Role-playing exercises will be used to explore appropriate options for dealing with challenging interpersonal situations.

The didactic sphere of skills pertinent to phlebotomy will also be addressed. Students will develop a concept for the rationale of each step in the procedures they perform. In addition, background information will be included in the discussion section of each lab. The rationale for procedural steps, quality control issues, safety issues, interpersonal skills, anatomy and physiology appropriate to the procedure, and historical perspectives will be discussed when appropriate.

The workbook is designed to be incorporated into a phlebotomy curriculum with a laboratory component. The workbook is structured to teach phlebotomy skills through a "layering" process. New information and techniques are introduced to the learner in a step-by-step process, which gradually acclimates the learner to the practice of phlebotomy.

Upon completion of the workbook, the students will have mastered standard phlebotomy procedures. The students' mastery of basic phlebotomy procedures will adequately prepare them to enter the clinical setting easily and effectively, requiring only minimal additional instruction. Optimally, after completing the workbook, the learner will be allowed to practice the techniques learned in a clinical setting.

It is assumed that the learner possesses at least a high school diploma but no background in the health care industry. Techniques presented are developed in stages, incorporating new concepts with each laboratory exercise. Each procedure is presented in the following format:

I. Patient interaction (approach, identification, explanation of procedure)
II. Preparation prior to a procedure (phlebotomist, equipment)
III. Site selection (skin puncture, venipuncture, arterial puncture)
IV. Site preparation (skin puncture, venipuncture, arterial puncture)
V. Postprocedure care
VI. Preparation of specimens for transport to the laboratory
VII. Appropriate disposal of waste materials

The quality of laboratory results is critically dependent on the quality of the specimen presented for analysis. Therefore, quality control, as it relates to the collection of specimens, is addressed in the workbook. The laboratory is equipped with very sophisticated and expensive instrumentation. Medical technologists and medical laboratory technicians are extensively trained to run analyses and interpret results. All of the technology and expertise available, however, can offer nothing if the blood specimen being analyzed was collected from the wrong patient. Patient identification and accurate labeling of patient specimens are particularly emphasized throughout the workbook.

The technique of specimen collection is critical to obtaining a quality specimen. Student performance of the laboratory exercises is assessed using a series of checklists. Most of the checklists include a subjective analysis of the student's performance, using the format "performed," "needs improvement," or "not performed" for each step of a given procedure. In some instances, the quality of the specimen generated is independent of the technique of specimen collection. For example, a variety of methods can generate a quality blood smear. In cases like blood smears, a checklist identifying acceptable characteristics of the specimen collected is provided. The instructor then indicates, via the checklist, the characteristics present or absent on a specimen submitted.

Finally, as a result of several years of teaching experience with students of phlebotomy, I recognized that certain teaching techniques were more effective than others. Specifically, I found that detailed direction was the most effective method of teaching phlebotomy techniques. Therefore, I have included comments related to my teaching experience that I hope will assist instructors and students in communicating the individual steps incorporated into basic phlebotomy skills.

General Safety Guidelines

What is a laboratory? *Webster's* dictionary defines a laboratory as follows: a building or room designed for scientific or technical investigation or experimentation; a situation or place providing the means for study, observation, or experimentation; a place where chemicals or medicines are prepared.

A clinical laboratory may be further defined as a building or room designed for the investigation and analyses of patient specimens. Patient specimens are analyzed for a variety of reasons, including: diagnosis of a clinical condition; monitoring a treatment regimen; isolation and identification of a suspected pathogen; susceptibility testing of a suspected pathogen; and compatibility testing prior to blood transfusion.

Laboratory analyses often involve reacting a patient's specimen with chemical reagents and measuring the results. Some elements of patient specimens may be measured using radioisotopes. The analyses are often performed by sophisticated and complex electronic instrumentation.

Inherent dangers are associated with working in an environment that incorporates the routine use of chemicals. Chemicals may be carcinogenic, caustic, corrosive, flammable, or poisonous. Radioisotopes present additional unique hazards associated with radioactive materials. Working in environments housing complex electronic instruments introduces all of the potential dangers associated with electricity. Finally, all of these situations present the inherent danger of fire.

These dangers could apply to any laboratory that uses chemicals, radioisotopes, and/or instruments to perform analyses. Since the clinical laboratory analyzes predominantly patient specimens, exposure to biohazardous materials is an additional potential risk.

To minimize the potential risks of working within the clinical laboratory, each laboratory should develop and implement safety policies and procedures. Everyone working in the laboratory should become familiar with the safety procedures established at that facility and follow them at all times.

General safety guidelines for the phlebotomist will be outlined and subsequently reflected in the laboratory exercises in this workbook. These guidelines are basic safety policies and procedures. Because policies and procedures vary from facility to facility, a supervisor should always be consulted for specific safety instructions.

Handwashing

Handwashing is the single most important procedure for preventing nosocomial infections. Handwashing is defined as a vigorous, brief rubbing together of all surfaces of lathered hands, followed by rinsing under a stream of water. Although various products are available, handwashing can be classified simply by whether plain soap or detergents or antimicrobial-containing products are used. Handwashing with plain soaps or detergents (in bar, granule, leaflet, or liquid form) suspends microorganisms and allows them to be rinsed off; this process is often referred to as mechanical removal of microorganisms. Handwashing with antimicrobial-containing products kills or inhibits the growth of microorganisms; this process is often referred to as chemical removal of microorganisms.

The microbial flora of the skin consists of resident and transient microorganisms. The resident microorganisms survive and multiply on the skin and can be repeatedly cultured, whereas the transient microbial flora represent recent contaminants that can survive only a limited period of time. Most resident microorganisms are found in superficial skin layers, but about 10% to 20% can inhabit deep epidermal layers. Handwashing with plain soaps and detergents is effective in removing many transient microbial flora. Resident microorganisms in the deep layers may not be removed by handwashing with plain soaps and detergents, but they usually can be killed or inhibited by handwashing with products that contain antimicrobial ingredients.

Phlebotomists should remove their gloves and wash their hands after EVERY blood collection procedure. Vigorous, brief rubbing together of all lathered surfaces for at least 10 seconds has been found to be effective in removing most microorganisms from the skin. When is it appropriate to use plain soap and when are antimicrobial soaps recommended for use? The absolute indications are not known due to a lack of well-defined studies in this area. This manual will incorporate the use of antimicrobial soaps in handwashing techniques. A specific step-by-step procedure to ensure thorough handwashing by persons learning the technique is developed in Lab #2.

Universal Precautions

Bloodborne pathogens are small organisms that may be present in the bloodstream, and they are capable of causing disease in humans. The 2 bloodborne pathogens that elicit the most concern are hepatitis B virus (HBV), which causes hepatitis B, and human immunodeficiency virus (HIV), which causes acquired immunodeficiency syndrome (AIDS).

The Centers for Disease Control (CDC) introduced the concept of universal precautions in 1983 to prevent the spread of bloodborne pathogens. Universal precautions are now mandated under the Occupational Safety and Health Administration's (OSHA) Bloodborne Pathogens Standard.

The term "universal precautions" refers to a system of infectious disease control. Under universal precautions, every direct contact with body fluids is considered potentially infectious. Universal precautions require every employee exposed to direct contact with body fluids to be protected as though such body fluids were infected with HBV or HIV. Therefore, universal precautions are intended to prevent health care workers from parenteral, mucous membrane, and non-intact skin exposures to bloodborne pathogens.

Under universal precautions introduced by CDC and now mandated by OSHA, phlebotomists must adhere to the following practices:

1. Wear gloves when performing blood collection procedures.
2. Wear protective gowns or lab coats when performing ANY type of blood collection procedure.

3. Dispose of ALL needles, lancets, and syringes in a needle disposal unit, appropriately labeled with the biohazard symbol.
4. Dispose of all other waste contaminated with blood or body fluids (including dried blood on gauze and bandage strips) in a red plastic bag marked with the biohazard symbol.

Personal Protective Equipment

Phlebotomists should wear gowns made of fluid-repellent material. The gowns may be worn from patient to patient, as long as they are not soiled. Once the gown becomes soiled, it should be changed immediately.

Phlebotomists must wear gloves for all blood collection procedures, including venipuncture, skin puncture, and arterial puncture. Gloves should fit appropriately and should be pulled up over the sleeves of the gown or lab coat. Gloves should be changed after EVERY patient. The phlebotomist should NEVER wash the gloves and wear them for subsequent patients, but they should be removed and discarded after every patient. After the gloves are removed, the hands should be washed.

Needle and Waste Disposal

Any object capable of puncturing a plastic bag (eg, needles, lancets, syringes) should be placed in a needle disposal unit. Needle disposal units are made of impenetrable plastic, making them a suitable disposal unit for sharp objects. All sharp objects must be placed in needle disposal units to prevent accidental puncture of staff by needles poking through a plastic bag.

Needles and other sharp objects should be placed in the needle disposal unit as soon as possible following a blood collection procedure. Needles should NEVER be recapped, bent, or broken.

Any waste materials contaminated with blood and/or body fluids that are not sharp should be discarded in a red plastic bag labeled with the biohazard symbol. Examples of this kind of waste material are gauze, cotton, or strip bandages contaminated with blood following a blood collection procedure.

Additional Precautions

In addition to collecting blood specimens from patients, the phlebotomist may be called upon to perform additional duties in the laboratory. This workbook instructs phlebotomists in some procedures that may or may not be routinely assigned to them, including microhematocrit determinations, ABO blood typing procedures, and blood smear preparations.

The OSHA Bloodborne Pathogens Standard has established engineering controls for these blood collection procedures. Please consult your supervisor about the safety policies and procedures associated with responsibilities of the phlebotomist within the clinical laboratory that are not blood specimen collection techniques.

Housekeeping

Phlebotomy chairs, the arms of phlebotomy chairs, and work surfaces should be cleaned with a disinfectant solution at the start of the shift, at the end of the shift, and as soon as any contamination occurs. An appropriate disinfectant is a 1:10 bleach solution (10 mL of bleach and 90 mL of water). For the disinfectant to be effective, the bleach solution must be prepared fresh daily.

If pieces of reusable equipment (tourniquets, needle holders) become contaminated, they must be cleaned immediately or discarded. Blood draw trays must be cleaned with an appropriate cleaning solution at least once a week, and more often if they become soiled.

Postpuncture Care

After collecting a blood specimen following skin puncture, place gauze over the puncture site. Instruct the patient to apply pressure. Inspect the site before leaving the patient. In adult patients only, if the site is still bleeding, apply a bandage over the puncture wound.

After withdrawing the needle after venipuncture, instruct the patient to apply pressure to the puncture site using the gauze that was placed over the site before needle withdrawal. The patient should keep his/her arm straight while applying pressure to minimize bruising. In adult patients only, if the site is still bleeding, apply a pressure bandage. Fold a 2 x 2-inch gauze square into fourths. Tape one edge of the bandage on one side of the puncture site. Pull the strip taut over the folded gauze and affix to the other side of the puncture.

First Aid

The following chart lists several of the most common adverse reactions a "patient" in the student phlebotomy lab may experience and the appropriate first aid to administer.

If any of these circumstances occur when performing the following laboratory exercises (or if any other abnormal circumstances not listed occur), notify the instructor or supervisor immediately.

Reaction	Symptoms	First Aid
Syncope (fainting)	Dizziness, weakness, pallor, clammy skin, sweating, unconsciousness	1) Release tourniquet 2) Remove needle 3) Elevate feet, loosen the collar, flex knees 4) Apply cold compress to back of the neck or forehead 5) Administer aromatic spirits of ammonia 6) Provide the donor with a cool beverage, such as orange juice
Nausea/vomiting	Pallor, clammy skin, sweating, dizziness, weakness	1) If the donor is only nauseated, instruct him/her to breathe slowly and deeply 2) Administer an emesis basin and towel, if necessary 3) Apply cold compress to the donor's forehead or the back of the neck
Hematoma at the puncture site	Purple color around the puncture site, swelling	1) Remove tourniquet 2) Remove needle 3) Elevate arm straight in the air, while applying pressure to the puncture site. Continue for at least 5 minutes 4) Apply ice or a cold pack to the puncture site for an additional 5 minutes 5) Apply a pressure bandage to the site 6) If the site is still swollen and/or painful, reapply the ice pack
Tetany	Deep and rapid respiration precedes the onset of muscular twitching and contractions, spasms of the ankles, wrists, and/or hands	Provide the donor with a paper bag and have him/her inhale and exhale with the bag placed over the mouth and nose

LAB 1

Values Clarification Techniques

Objective

To develop characteristics consistent with the term "professionalism"; to rank these professional characteristics according to their significance; to internalize the concept of professionalism in terms of a personal value set

Equipment

Worksheets;
Pen or pencil;
Personal "value set"

Directions: Follow the instructions given on each values clarification technique. After everyone has completed the worksheets, the instructor will lead a discussion about the issues raised by the exercises.

Please note: There are no correct or incorrect answers. Students are to respond to the questions using their own value set. Some of the exercises clearly have no desirable answer and are designed in this manner to motivate the student to differentiate the corresponding values of the characteristics presented.

Students should begin to develop a hierarchy of values that will ultimately become their personal concept of professionalism. Once the hierarchy of values is defined and internalized, students will begin to behave consistently with their internalized value system, which, in turn, is consistent with their concept of professionalism.

Exercise 1

Directions: Using numbers 1 to 11, rank the characteristics listed below in order of importance, relative to *your* concept of a professional appearance. Award #1 to the most important characteristic and #11 to the least important characteristic. Use each number one time only.

______1. Conservative dress

______2. Cleanliness

______3. Ironed clothes

______4. Clean, closed-toe shoes

______5. Clean, confined hair

______6. Trimmed beards and moustaches

______7. Clean hands

______8. Groomed nails

______9. Limited amounts of jewelry

______10. Undetectable body odor

______11. Fresh breath

Exercise 2

Directions: Listed below are 10 questions with several alternate choices. Rank each choice according to your own value system. Award #1 to the highest-ranking choice and #3 (or #4) to the lowest-ranking choice. The numbers may be used only once for each question.

1. Which of the following persons would you prefer to draw your blood?

______An incompetent phlebotomist who appears very professional

______A very competent phlebotomist who appears unprofessional

______A very competent phlebotomist who appears very professional

2. Rank the characteristics below from most professional to least professional.

______Unhurried manner

______Considerate manner

______Gentle manner

3. Rank the professional characteristics below from most important to least important.

______Honesty

______Confidentiality

______Appearance

______Competency

4. **Rank the grooming characteristics below from most important to least important.**

______Clean clothes

______Conservative clothes

______Groomed nails

5. **A phlebotomist is going to interact with a patient for the first time. Rank the following characteristics according to how each would instill the most confidence in the patient.**

______Competency (phlebotomist is certified with several years of experience)

______Appearance (phlebotomist is well groomed and follows the facility's dress code)

______Attitude (phlebotomist is pleasant and unhurried)

6. **Rank the following actions from most consistent with the concept of professional to least consistent with this concept.**

______Chewing gum noisily

______Lighting a cigarette in the patients' lounge

______Listening to personal stereo headphones on the way to drawing blood

7. **Rank the following appearances from most consistent with the concept of professional to least consistent with this concept.**

______Dirty lab coat

______Untrimmed beard

______Dirty hands

8. Rank the following demeanors from most consistent with the concept of professional to least consistent with this concept.

______A phlebotomist "in a hurry"

______A phlebotomist who insists on drawing a patient's blood while the patient is in the middle of a bed bath

______A phlebotomist who rapidly pulls down an elderly patient's arm to position it properly for venipuncture

9. Rank the following behaviors from most consistent with the concept of professional to least consistent with this concept.

______The phlebotomist who "makes up" results to a Duke bleeding time test

______The phlebotomist who sees her neighbor in the psychiatric department and tells her bridge club (all neighbors) about it that night

______The phlebotomist who pulls her wrinkled lab coat out of the bottom of her locker and puts it on before leaving for the floor

10. Rank the following phlebotomists according to the kind of image that is projected to the patients about the laboratory and the hospital.

______An incompetent phlebotomist who appears very professional

______A very competent phlebotomist who appears very unprofessional

______A very competent phlebotomist who appears very professional

Exercise 3

Directions: Below is a line representing a continuum. Place each of the following life experiences on the continuum.

A. Job	B. Family	C. School	D. Household duties
E. Sleep	F. Entertainment	G. Leisure time	

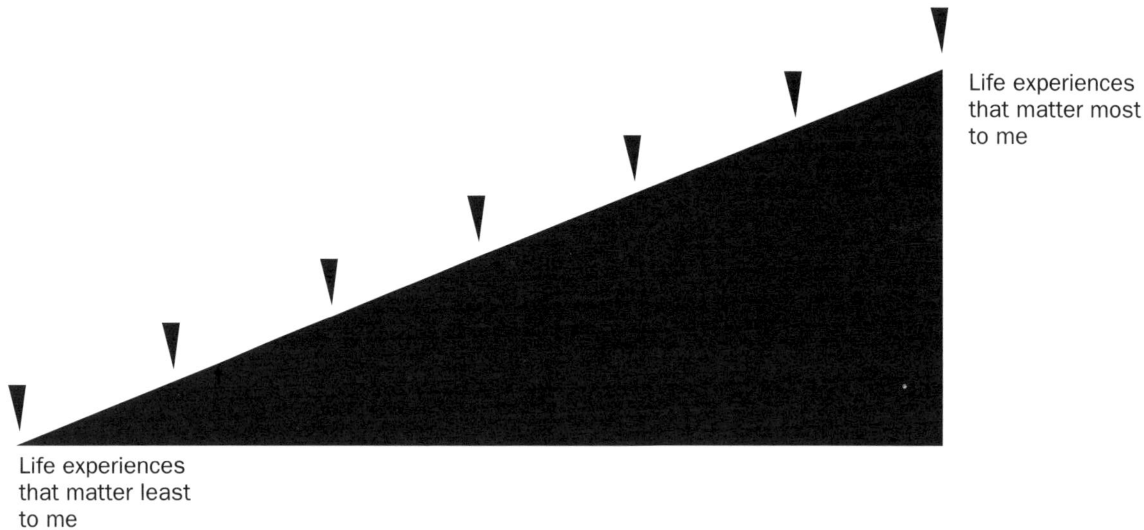

LAB 2

Handwashing Procedures

Objective

To familiarize the student with handwashing procedures appropriate for the clinical laboratory

Equipment

Antiseptic soap;
Paper towels;
Running water

Discussion

As phlebotomists perform routine daily activities in the laboratory, their hands may come in contact with body fluids potentially capable of containing pathogenic organisms. As a result, a phlebotomist's hands are capable of acting as a vector in the transmission of infections. Frequent handwashing is essential to preventing the spread of infection, both to the phlebotomist and to any patients the phlebotomist may encounter.

Hands should be washed at the following times:

- When visibly contaminated with blood, body fluids, or tissues
- After every patient contact
- After removal of gloves and other protective wear or equipment
- Before leaving the clinical work areas
- Before eating, drinking, smoking, applying makeup, or changing contact lenses outside of the lab, and after using lavatory facilities
- Before all other activities that entail hand contact with mucous membranes or a break in the skin
- Periodically during the day when routinely handling and testing body fluids

Rings and bracelets should not be worn because they might interfere with a thorough handwashing. They also make it more difficult to don gloves.

Frequent handwashing can be very damaging to the skin's normal protective mechanisms by damaging or cracking skin, altering its pH, or changing its normal flora. Application of hand lotion may reduce this damage; lab personnel, therefore, are encouraged to use it. The use of hand lotion is restricted, however, and it should not be applied in the following circumstances: immediately after washing one's hands; immediately before giving direct patient care; and immediately before handling sensitive instruments or equipment. Lotions might interfere with the residual action of antimicrobial handwashing products.

Procedure:

Handwashing

1. Release some paper toweling from the dispenser. (This step is only appropriate if the towels are contained on a roll within a canister dispenser.)
2. Turn the water faucet on. Adjust the temperature to a comfortable level.
3. Dispense a small amount of soap (3–5 mL) into the palm of the hand.
4. Create a lather, using the soap (**Fig. 2-1**). Use as much friction as needed to remove gross contamination and dead skin (**Fig. 2-2**).
5. Rinse the soap off the hands. Be sure to hold the hands in a downward position. Allow the water to run off the hands and into the sink (**Fig. 2-3**).
6. Redispense a small amount of soap into the palm of the hand. Create a lather, using the soap. During this step, pay attention to cleansing the fingernails and nail beds.
7. Using the thumb of one hand, gently rub around the cuticle and nail bed of each finger and thumb of the opposite hand (**Fig. 2-4**). Repeat this step, alternating hands.

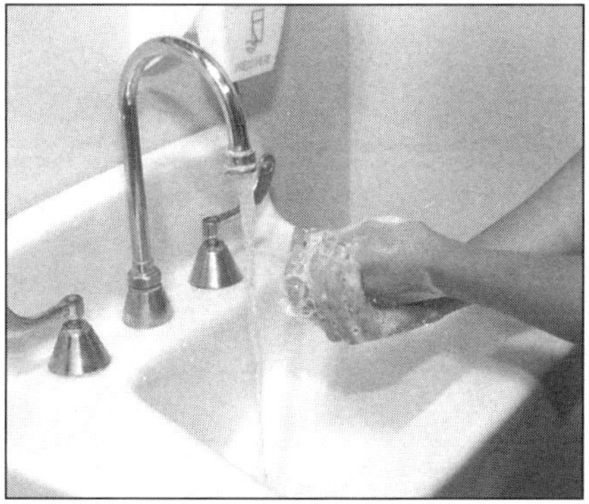

Figure 2-1 Create an adequate lather.

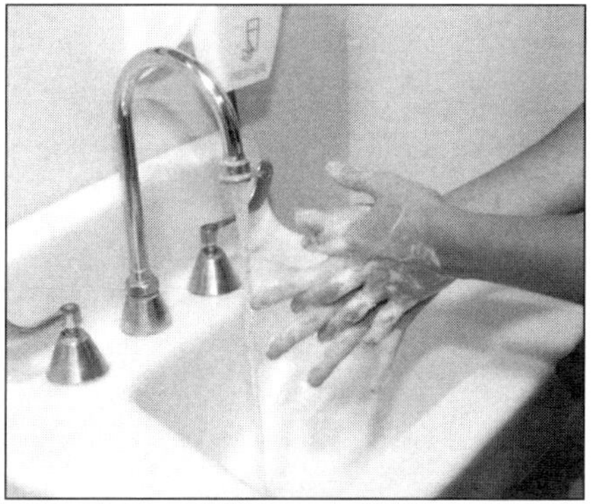

Figure 2-2 Use friction to remove contamination.

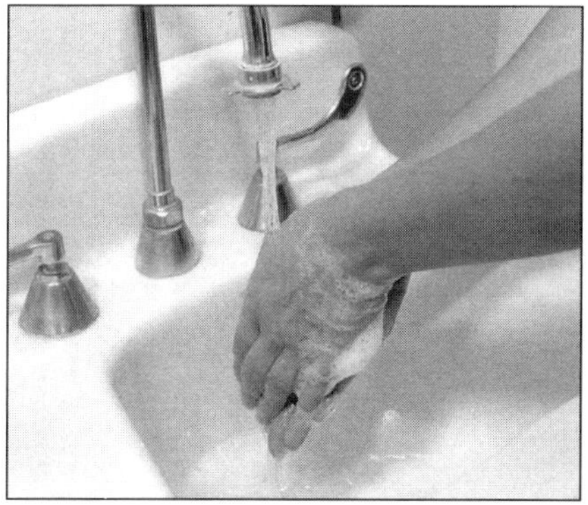

Figure 2-3 Rinse in a downward position.

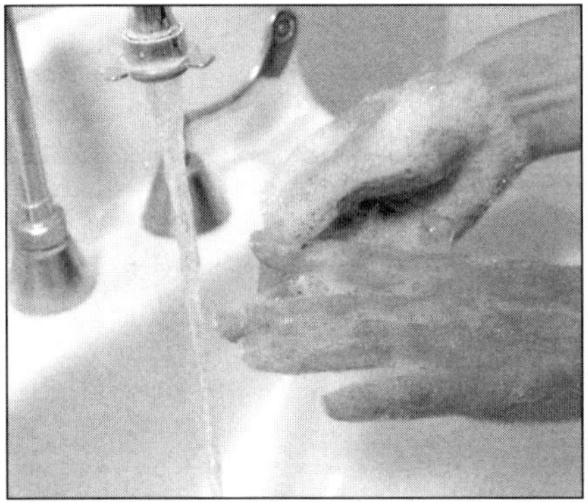

Figure 2-4 Use thumb to clean cuticles.

8. Be sure to clean underneath the nails (on the palmar surface of the hand). To accomplish this, the phlebotomist may:

a. Rub the nails of one hand across the palm of the other hand, creating a friction sufficient to clean underneath the nails (**Fig. 2-5**). Repeat this step, alternating hands. This method is recommended for persons with short nails.

b. If a person has long nails, it is appropriate to take the nail of one finger, usually the index finger or the thumb, and use it to clean beneath each nail on the opposite hand (**Fig. 2-6**). Repeat this procedure, alternating hands.

9. Rinse the hands under running water, being sure to hold the hands in a downward position (see **Fig. 2-3**).

10. Use paper toweling to thoroughly dry the hands.

11. Using the same piece of paper towel, turn off the water supply (**Fig. 2-7**). DO NOT touch the faucet handles with your hands once they have been washed.

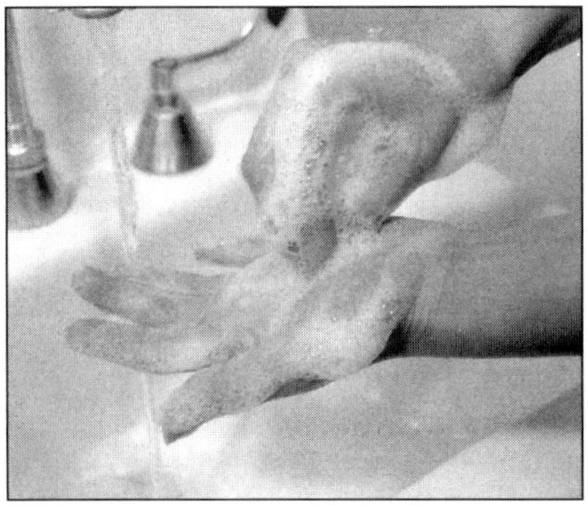

Figure 2-5 Rub nails across palm of the hand.

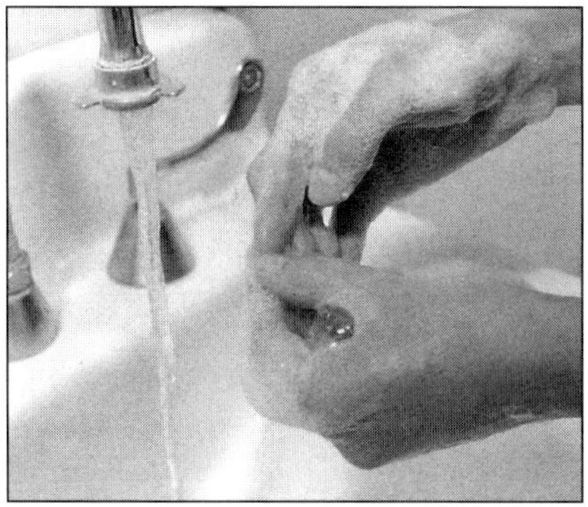

Figure 2-6 Use left thumbnail to clean under nails on the right hand.

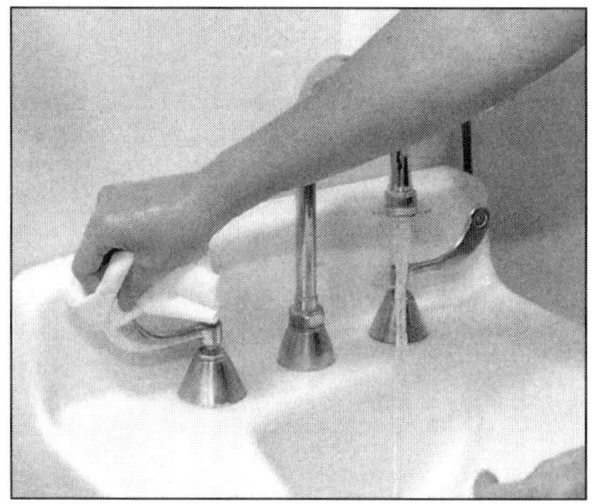

Figure 2-7 Use paper towel to turn off water.

Checklist:
Handwashing

(A) Performed **(B) Needs Improvement** **(C) Not Performed**

Comments:

______ 1. Positions paper towel.
______ 2. Turns water supply on.
______ 3. Adjusts water temperature.
______ 4. Dispenses an appropriate amount of soap into the hand.
______ 5. Creates a sufficient amount of lather.
______ 6. Sufficiently removes gross contamination from the skin surface.
______ 7. Rinses off soap.
______ 8. Appropriately positions hands while rinsing them.
______ 9. Redispenses soap into the palm of the hand.
______ 10. Cleanses the nail beds of each finger.
______ 11. Cleanses underneath the nails in an appropriate fashion.
______ 12. Rinses off soap.
______ 13. Appropriately positions hands while rinsing.
______ 14. Dries hands, using paper towels.
______ 15. Uses paper towel to turn off water supply.

Study Questions
Lab 2

1. Define the following terms:

Antiseptic: ______________________________

Disinfectant: ______________________________

Quarternary ammonia compounds: ______________________________

2. Give 2 examples of each of these solutions:

Antiseptic: ______________________________

____

Disinfectant: ______________________________

____

Quarternary ammonia compound: ______________________________

____

3. Define nosocomial infection: ______________________________

____

4. List 3 types of patients most susceptible to nosocomial infections:

____

____

____

LAB 3

Gowning, Gloving, & Masking

Objective

To properly don and remove the protective clothing required in isolation procedures

Equipment

Antiseptic soap; Running water; Paper towels; Gowns, Masks, Gloves; 3 Blood agar plates; 2 Sterile swabs; 37°C Incubator

Discussion

Isolating patients within the hospital for infection control is usually done for one of the following reasons:

1. To minimize the risk of transmitting infectious agents from the patient to persons in contact with the patient;
2. To protect patients who are extremely susceptible to infections, usually as a result of a weakened immune system.

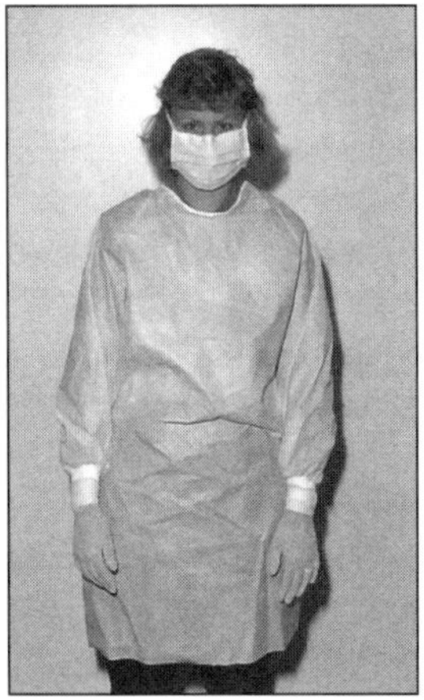

Figure 3-1 Appropriate protective clothing for approaching patients in strict isolation.

There are several classifications of isolation. The type of protective clothing required for each category has been established by the Centers for Disease Control. Before entering the room of a patient in isolation, health care workers should consult the sign on the patient's door. The sign will detail which articles of protective clothing are required. After washing their hands, health care workers should don the articles of protective clothing specified before entering the patient's room.

This demonstration will address the protective clothing required for entering rooms of patients in strict isolation. Patients in strict isolation have highly communicable diseases that may be spread by direct contact, indirect contact, and airborne droplets. Health care workers approaching patients in strict isolation must wear gowns, gloves, and masks (**Fig. 3-1**).

Demonstration

This exercise will demonstrate the presence of unseen organisms in the student laboratory or work environment.

1. Inspect the 3 blood agar culture plates to ensure that no organisms are present.
2. Label the first blood agar plate "faucet."
3. Run the cotton tip of the sterile swab over several surfaces of the faucet.
4. Roll the sterile swab onto the blood agar. Then gently move the swab back and forth over the blood agar.
5. Label the second blood agar plate "air."
6. Remove the cover of the dish and allow the room air to interact with the blood agar for at least 5 minutes. Replace the cover.
7. Label the third blood agar plate "hand."
8. Ask a volunteer to place the fingerprints of both the right and left hands onto the blood agar. Take a sterile swab and gently move it across the fingerprints on the agar.
9. Incubate all 3 culture plates at 37°C.
10. Inspect for growth at 24 and 48 hours. Bacterial growth will occur in the form of colonies, which will appear as round spots, usually white or yellow, on the surface of the blood agar plate.

Usually, growth will occur on all 3 plates after 48 hours of incubation at 37°C. This demonstration dramatically illustrates the presence of microscopic organisms. The rationale for placing patients in isolation is to prevent the transmission of microorganisms and, thus, break the cycle of infectivity.

Procedure 1:

Donning Protective Clothing

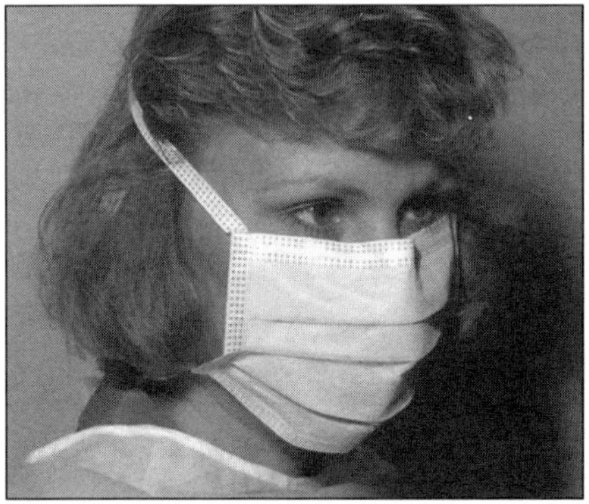

Figure 3-2 Mask fits securely over nose and mouth.

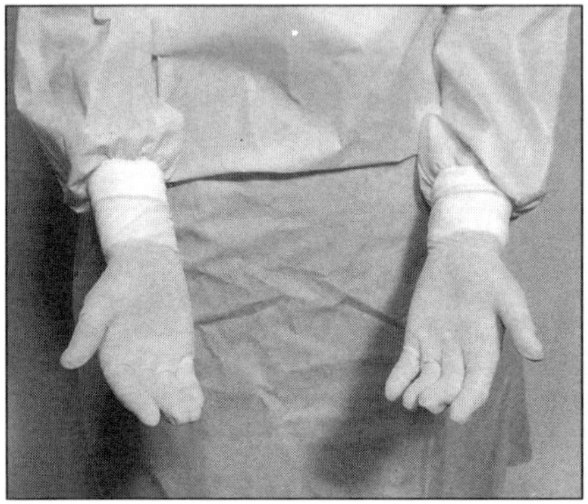

Figure 3-3 Cuffs of the gloves are pulled up over sleeves of gown.

1. Wash hands (refer to Lab #2).
2. Remove lab coat. Pick up the gown from the inside, near the openings for the arms. Let it fall open, but do not allow it to touch the floor. Put one arm in and then the other, so the opening is in the back.
3. Tie the neck strings and then the waistband.
4. Determine which side of the mask should be placed next to the face. Some masks have the inside marked "inside." Other masks are manufactured with the outside of the mask a different color than the inside. It is important that masks are donned with the appropriate side out so the filtering system of the mask is operational.
5. Put on the mask, making sure the outside of the mask is to the outside of your body. Masks usually have a piece of wire (similar to the twist ties used to fasten bags) at the top of the mask. Bend the wire to fit snugly over the bridge of your nose (**Fig. 3-2**).
6. Tie the ties high on your head and above the ears. Be sure to tie them securely, so the mask does not slip off.
7. Put on the gloves. Be sure the cuff of the glove is pulled up over the sleeve of the gown (**Fig. 3-3**).

Procedure 2:

Removing Isolation Clothing

1. Untie the gown at the waist (**Fig. 3-4**).
2. Slip a finger from one hand underneath the cuff of the glove on the opposite hand (**Fig. 3-5**).
3. Pull the glove off, turning it inside out as it is removed (**Fig. 3-6**).
4. Deposit in the designated waste receptacle. Repeat the procedure on the opposite hand.
5. Remove the mask by untying the ties. Be careful not to touch the front of the mask (**Fig. 3-7**). Holding the mask by the ties, deposit in the designated waste receptacle (**Fig. 3-8**).

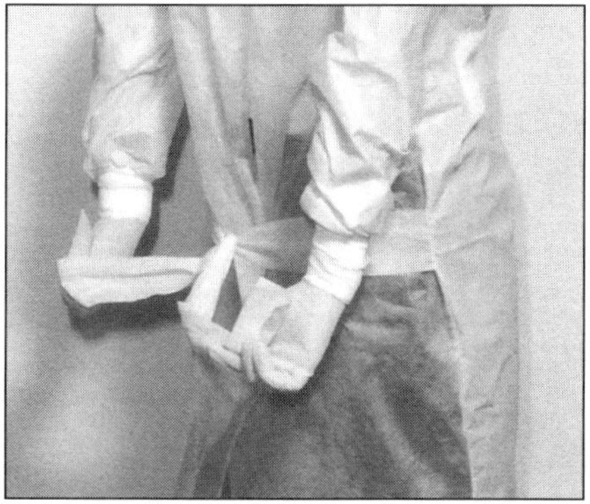

Figure 3-4 Untie gown at waist.

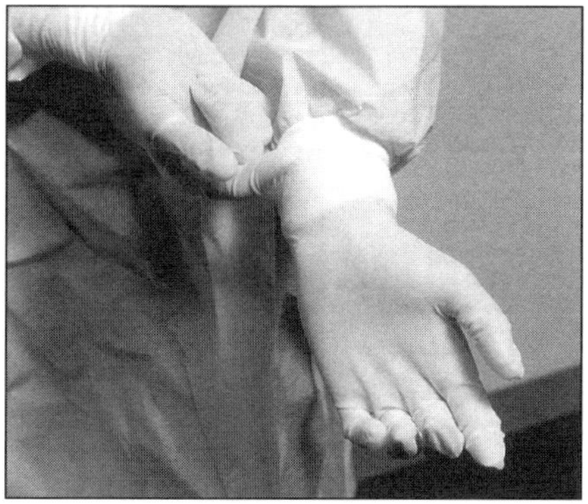

Figure 3-5 Slip finger underneath the cuff of the glove to remove.

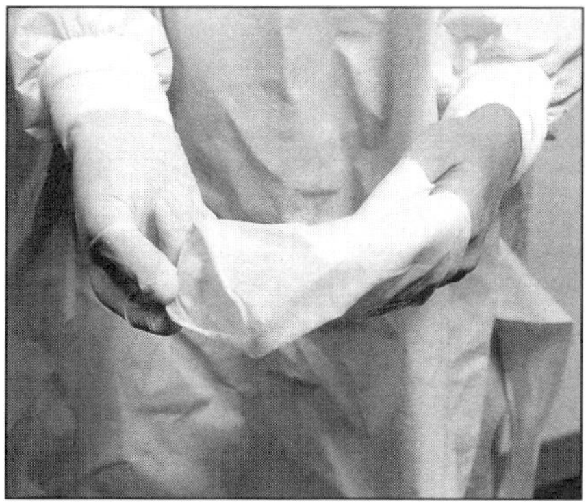

Figure 3-6 Turn glove inside out as it is removed.

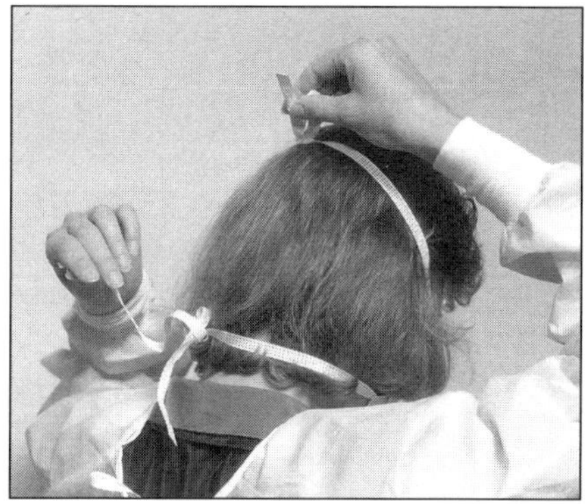

Figure 3-7 Untie mask without touching the front.

6. Untie the tie at the neck of the gown (**Fig. 3-9**). Using the ties, pull the gown down toward the front of the body.
7. Pull one arm out of its sleeve, turning the sleeve inside out as you proceed. Repeat, using the other arm (**Fig. 3-10**). Be sure the front of the gown does not contact your hands or uniform! Deposit the gown in the designated waste receptacle.
8. Wash hands before proceeding to the next patient.
9. Don lab coat (removed at the beginning of this procedure).

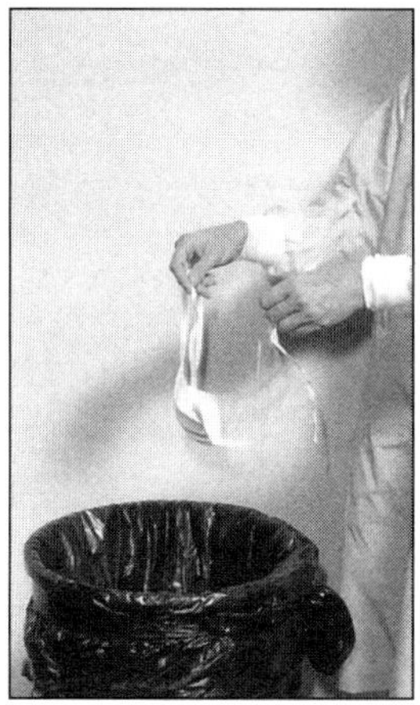

Figure 3-8 Hold mask by ties when disposing.

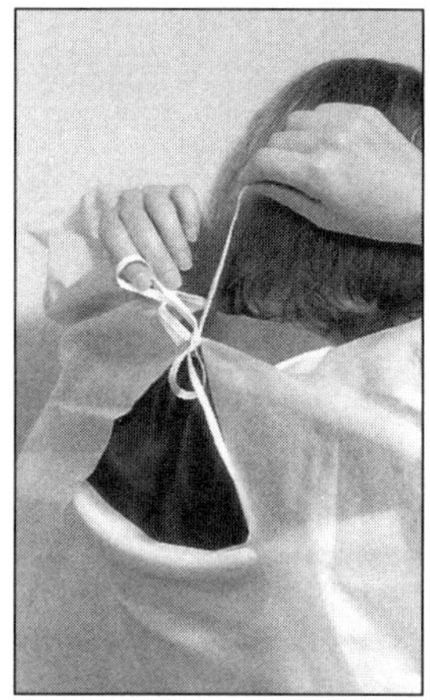

Figure 3-9 Untie gown at neck.

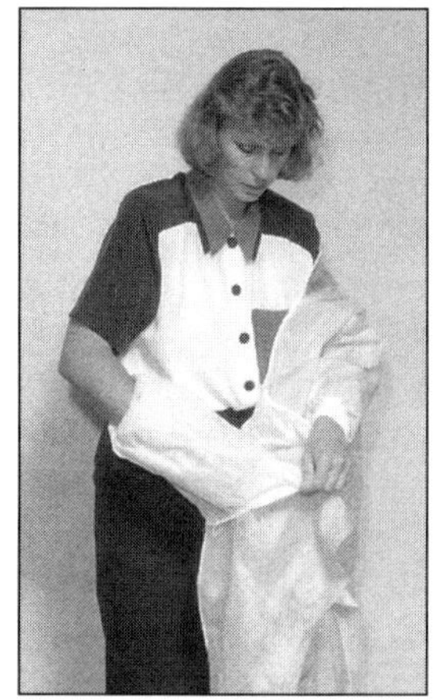

Figure 3-10 Turn gown inside out as it is removed.

Checklist: Gowning, Gloving, & Masking

(A) Performed **(B) Needs Improvement** **(C) Not Performed**

Comments:

______ 1. Removes lab coat.
______ 2. Washes hands before putting on the protective clothing.
______ 3. Dons gown, tying the ties at the neck and waist.
______ 4. Dons mask.
______ 5. Positions mask with the appropriate side facing out.
______ 6. Securely fastens the wire at the top of the mask around the nose.
______ 7. Securely ties the ties high on the head.
______ 8. Dons gloves.
______ 9. Positions gloves so the cuff is pulled over the sleeve of the gown.
______ 10. Unties gown first at the waist to remove the protective clothing.
______ 11. Removes gloves.
______ 12. Removes gloves inside out.
______ 13. Deposits gloves in the appropriate receptacle.
______ 14. Removes mask.
______ 15. Only touches the ties when removing the mask.
______ 16. Deposits mask in the appropriate receptacle.
______ 17. Unties gown at the neck.
______ 18. Removes gown inside out.
______ 19. Does not touch the front of the gown with either the hands or uniform during removal.
______ 20. Washes hands before continuing on to next patient.

Study Questions
Lab 3

1. Define universal precautions: ____________________

____

2. Describe the infection control chain: ____________________

____

3. List 4 ways infectious disease agents are transmitted: ____________________

____

4. Draw the biohazard symbol:

5. Draw the radiation symbol:

6. Draw the National Fire Protection Association (NFPA) hazard sign:

7. Describe the NFPA hazard rating system. How does this system relate to the NFPA hazard sign? ____________________

____

8. What are the 3 principles of protecting oneself from radiation exposure? _____

____

____

LAB 4

Quality Control/Equipment

Objective

To introduce the concepts of quality assurance and quality control; to familiarize the student with quality control procedures associated with equipment commonly incorporated into routine phlebotomy procedures

Equipment

Unopened box of sterile evacuated tubes; Unopened box of EDTA (or other anticoagulant) evacuated tubes; Sterile swab; Blood agar culture plate; 37°C incubator; Gauze; Centrifuge; Stopwatch; Tachometer; Calibrated aneroid gauge; Gown, Gloves; Mask

Discussion

Quality assurance is a term used to denote a program that guarantees quality patient care. Quality assurance applies to the totality of patient care. Quality assurance in the clinical laboratory is implemented when a program is in place to monitor the following situations:

1. Patient preparation
2. Specimen collection
3. Specimen transportation
4. Specimen processing
5. Instrumental and technical performance of laboratory tests
6. Laboratory safety
7. In-service training and education of laboratory workers

Quality control is a term used to denote specific procedures within a quality assurance program designed to ensure quality patient care.

Quality control procedures minimize or control variation inherent in testing procedures so that fluctuations in results are caused by changes in the patient's condition and not by changes in the testing methods. Quality control procedures attempt to standardize as much of the test procedure as possible. "Standardize" means to perform a particular procedure exactly the same way every time. "Standardize" also means that every individual will perform a particular procedure exactly the same way (ie, 2 persons performing the same procedure will arrive at identical results). Standardization of laboratory analyses begins with blood collection procedures. Therefore, of the 7 categories of quality assurance, the phlebotomist is most closely associated with patient preparation, specimen collection, and specimen transport.

Quality Control
Patient Preparation

Quality test results depend heavily on quality patient preparation. Patient preparation refers to procedures patients must follow before having their blood drawn. Strict adherence to preparation procedures is critical to quality test results.

If the patient is an inpatient, the nursing service will oversee patient preparation. If the patient is an outpatient, laboratory personnel, and many times the phlebotomist, will provide patient preparation instructions.

The phlebotomist plays a critical role in ensuring adequate and appropriate patient care. The phlebotomist may interview the patient to ensure the patient's adherence to preparatory guidelines. If the phlebotomist discovers that the patient did not appropriately follow the preparation guidelines for a particular test, he or she must inform the supervisor about the situation.

The most common example of patient preparation is fasting, which means the patient refrains from eating for at least 8 hours before the blood is collected. The specimen taken is referred to as a "fasting" specimen. Specific patient preparation procedures will be discussed with specific specimen collection techniques.

Quality Control
Specimen Transport

Once a specimen has been collected, it must be transported to the laboratory. It is important that the specimen arrive in the laboratory in a timely fashion following collection to ensure quality results. Blood constituents undergo chemical and morphologic changes over time. If a sufficient amount of time passes, the changes can be clinically significant and incorrectly indicate a change in the patient's condition. Transport guidelines vary from specimen to specimen (see Appendix 2).

Quality Control

Evacuated Tubes

Patient blood specimens are collected into evacuated tubes (**Fig. 4-1**). Evacuated tube manufacturers are responsible for evaluating the tubes before shipping to ensure that the tubes adhere to quality control standards generally accepted in the field. However, when a shipment of tubes is received from the manufacturer, the phlebotomy department is responsible for assessing the quality of the tubes prior to use.

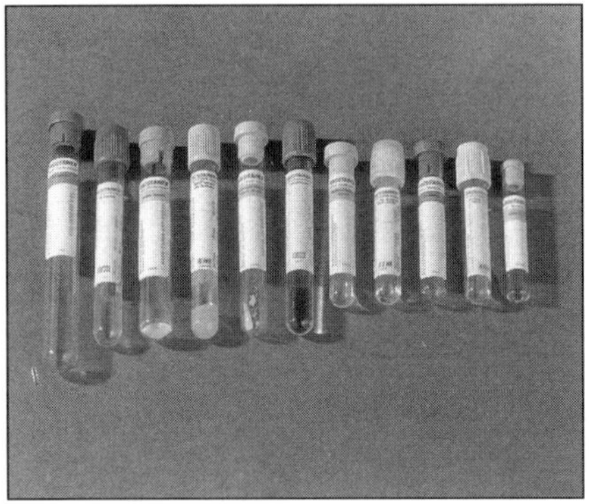

Figure 4-1 Various sizes of evacuated tubes.

Tubes are manufactured according to "lots." Each lot, or batch, of tubes is assigned a lot number. A sample of tubes from a particular lot number is assessed, and the results of that assessment are generally applied to the entire lot number. In other words, if a few tubes in a particular lot are found to be acceptable for use, it can be assumed that the rest of the tubes from that lot number are also acceptable for use.

In addition to a lot number, each batch of tubes is assigned an expiration date. Evacuated tubes should not be used to collect blood specimens beyond the designated expiration date because the additive may lose its reactivity, thus rendering the specimen inappropriate for testing. The tube may also lose some of its vacuum after the expiration date, which may result in the tube drawing less blood than the volume specified, altering the blood:additive ratio in the tube. If the excess additive in the tube is liquid, it will dilute the blood specimen. Consequently, laboratory results may be erroneously decreased due to inappropriate specimen collection and not as a result of a change in the patient's condition.

Every time a new box of tubes is opened for use, the expiration date should be noted. If the tubes have exceeded the expiration date, they should not be used to collect patient specimens.

Evacuated tubes are generally inspected for the following: gross manufacturing defects; sterility; durability; volume of draw (refer to Lab #5); appropriate functioning of additive; and expiration date.

Quality Control

Centrifuges

A centrifuge is an instrument that separates the lighter portions of a mixture from the heavier portions of a mixture by centrifugal force. Centrifugal force is the force exerted on an object when the object is moved in a circle. Centrifuges are equipped with holders or carriers for blood specimens (**Fig. 4-2**). The arm holding the carriers spins the blood specimens around at a predetermined rate, defined as rotations per minute, or RPMs.

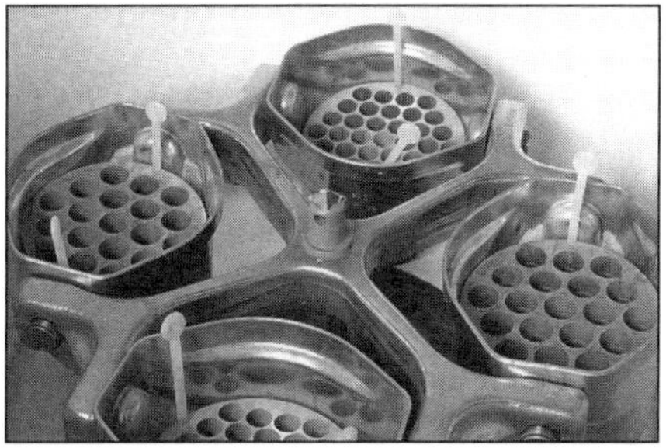

Figure 4-2 Centrifuge holders for specimens.

Centrifuges are available in a wide variety of sizes to accommodate a wide variety of blood volumes. Specimens are placed in a centrifuge during processing to separate the fluid portion of the blood from the cellular portion. Varying the number of RPMs or the length of time a specimen is centrifuged will alter the density of the cellular component packed at the bottom of the tube. To ensure uniform processing of specimens, the RPMs and timing device must be checked periodically to be sure both are operating within acceptable parameters.

Quality Control

Blood Pressure Cuffs

Sphygmomanometers (blood pressure cuffs) are used for certain phlebotomy procedures, specifically the modified Ivy template bleeding time and for blood pressure determinations during donor screening procedures. Blood pressure cuffs must be evaluated on a regular basis to ensure standardized readings.

Quality Control

Equipment

The focus of this lab will be quality control procedures designed to ensure the quality of equipment used for routine phlebotomy procedures. Quality control of equipment is the first step toward quality specimen collection because it is performed in the laboratory before the equipment is used to ensure its suitability. Equipment used by phlebotomists in the clinical laboratory is usually evaluated on a regular basis, with each piece being evaluated on a different schedule. The schedules for maintenance checks on equipment vary from facility to facility. Usually, the schedules established adhere to College of American Pathologists (CAP) or Joint Commission on Accreditation of Healthcare Organizations (JCAHO) guidelines for equipment quality control.

Procedure 1: Quality Control/ Evacuated Tubes

For each new lot number of tubes, the phlebotomist should:

1. Don gown, gloves, and mask.
2. Visually inspect for the presence of additives and foreign materials, such as glass chips and stopper material. Such materials occasionally appear in evacuated tubes due to manufacturing defects.
3. If the tubes selected for use have sterile interiors, 2 tubes from the new lot number should be cultured to ensure the sterility of the interior of the tubes.
   A. Remove the stopper from one of the evacuated tubes.
   B. Using a sterile swab, swab the inside of the tube opened. Roll the swab around the interior of the tube.
   C. Open a blood agar Petri dish. Rub the swab across the agar. Replace the cover of the Petri dish. Label the dish "tube."
   D. Place the Petri dish in a 37°C incubator.
   E. Monitor the agar plates for growth. If the blood collection tubes are not sterile, colonies will appear on the culture plate. Colonies will appear as round spots, usually white or pale yellow in color, on the surface of the blood agar in the dish. If the tubes are sterile, there will not be any growth on the agar plates. Most facilities monitor the culture plates for at least 48 hours. Some facilities will use the sterile swab to inoculate thioglycolate broth. Thioglycolate broth is observed for growth over 7 days.
4. Have the instructor fill 2 evacuated tubes with blood via venipuncture. Place the tubes in the centrifuge. Centrifuge the filled tubes for 10 minutes at the recommended number of RPMs for the equipment you are using.
   A. Check the tubes for durability during centrifugation. (Are they cracked or broken following centrifugation?)
   B. Check the tubes for stopper removal immediately following centrifugation. (Did the stoppers pop off the tubes prematurely?)
5. Evacuated tubes should be checked for accuracy associated with the volume of draw. (This aspect of quality control will be addressed in Lab #5.)

6. The effectiveness of anticoagulant in evacuated tubes should be evaluated. For example, a blood specimen should be collected by venipuncture into an EDTA tube. The blood should be poured through a gauze. The gauze should be inspected for clots. Blood specimens collected in EDTA are most often used for hematology testing. A large portion of testing performed in the hematology department is cell counting. Most automated methods of cell counting will be compromised if the specimen contains clots. Therefore, it is important that EDTA tubes be effective in preventing clot formation.
7. Evacuated tubes should also be evaluated for metals contamination. This methodology, however, is beyond the scope of the phlebotomy student lab and, therefore, will not be addressed in this workbook.

Procedure 2: Quality Control/ Needles

1. Check the needle box to ensure an acceptable expiration date.
2. Prior to use, all needles should be visually inspected to be sure the seal is intact. Any needle with a broken or suspect seal should be appropriately discarded. This practice should be adhered to prior to EVERY venipuncture.
3. Immediately after the cap has been removed from the needle, visually inspect the needle for burrs, hooks, or other signs of manufacturing error (**Fig. 4-3**). If a needle has a hook or a burr or appears otherwise unsuitable, the needle should be discarded and a new one opened for use.

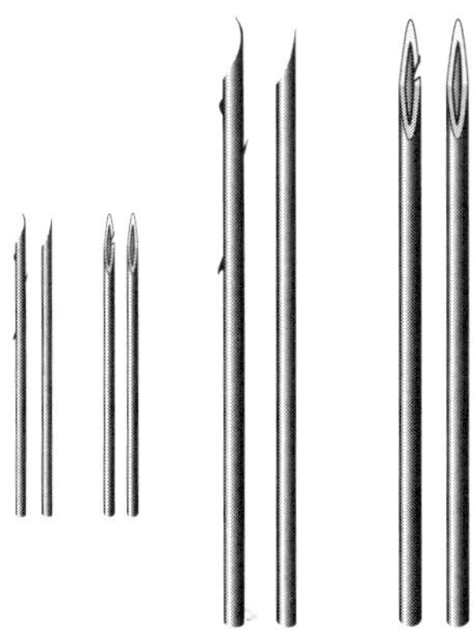

Figure 4-3 The 2 small pairs of needles on the left are actual size; those on the right are enlarged. In each pair, the needle on the left is unacceptable, the one on the right is acceptable.

Procedure 3: Quality Control/ Centrifuges

1. Using an acceptably standardized stopwatch, compare the accuracy of the timing device on the centrifuge with the standardized stopwatch (**Fig. 4-4**).
2. Using a tachometer, measure the RPMs of your centrifuge model (**Fig. 4-5**). Your instructor will provide you with instructions for the tachometer used at your facility and will give you the acceptable ranges for tachometer readings for the centrifuge used at your facility.

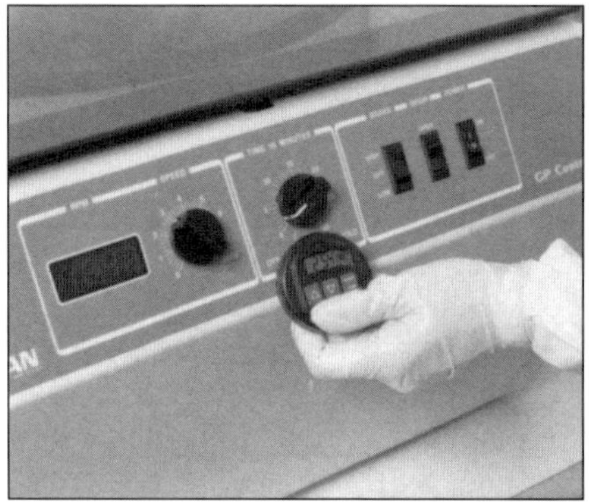

Figure 4-4 Use a stopwatch to compare accuracy of the timing device of the centrifuge.

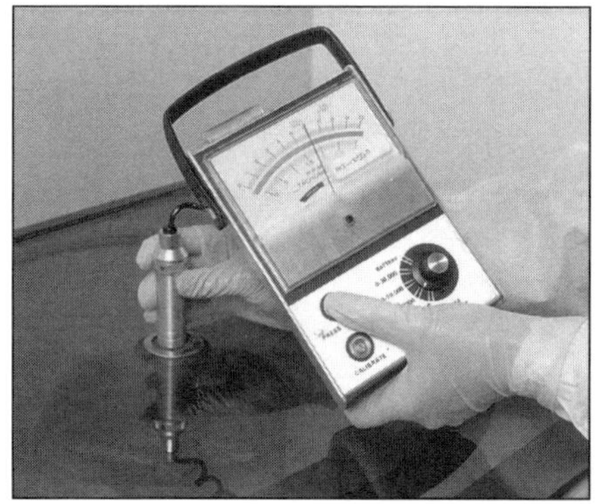

Figure 4-5 Use a tachometer to measure the RPMs of the centrifuge.

Procedure 4:

Quality Control/ Blood Pressure Cuff

Accuracy Checks for Sphygmomanometers*

Sphygmomanometers should be checked at least quarterly.

1. The aneroid gauge is guaranteed to be accurate throughout the scale as long as it is within the "0" reading in the absence of pressure. If ever out of "0," the gauge should be returned to the factory for repair and recalibration.
2. The inflating system, exhaust valve, and tubing should be checked for leaks in pressure. These leaks should not exceed more than 5 mm Hg/sec. Inflate cuff to 250 mm Hg. Hold the pressure for 1 minute to test for slow leaks.
3. Test the gauge for accuracy against a calibrated gauge. Position the cuff around a cylinder. Pump air into the cuff until the dial reads 100 mm Hg (**Fig. 4-6**). Clamp the tube leading to the gauge so that it is airtight. When air is unable to escape, remove the gauge from the tube and insert the calibrated gauge in its place (**Fig. 4-7**). Unclamp the tube. Both gauges should read the same pressure (**Fig. 4-8**). A difference of more than 5 mm Hg is unacceptable. The gauge in question should be returned to the factory for recalibration.

*Adapted with permission. Garza D, Becan-McBride K. *Phlebotomy Handbook*. East Norwalk, Conn: Appleton and Lange; 1989:243.

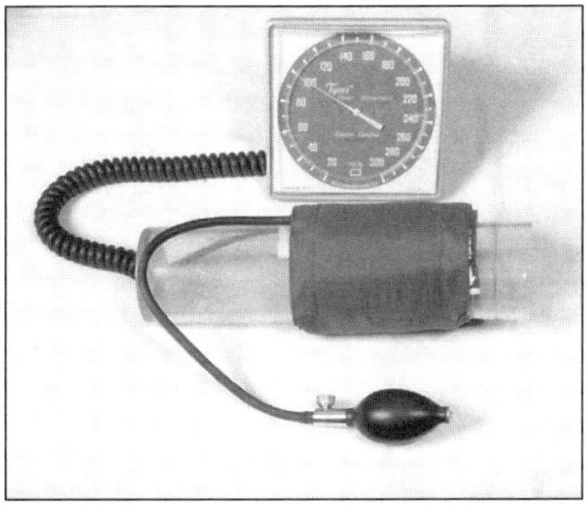

Figure 4-6 Pump air into the cuff until the dial reads 100 mm Hg.

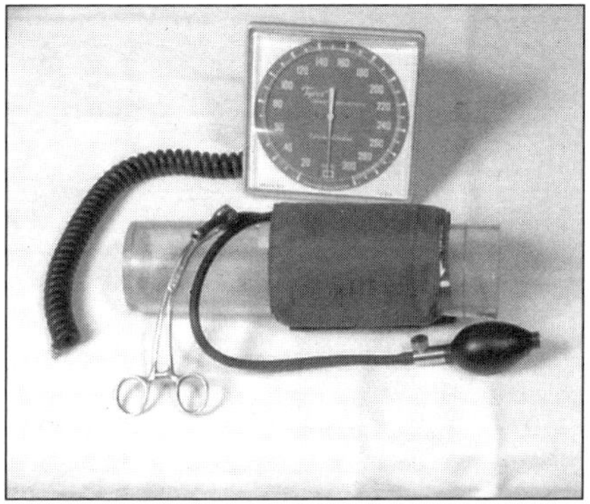

Figure 4-7 Clamp the tube, remove the first gauge, and insert the calibrated gauge.

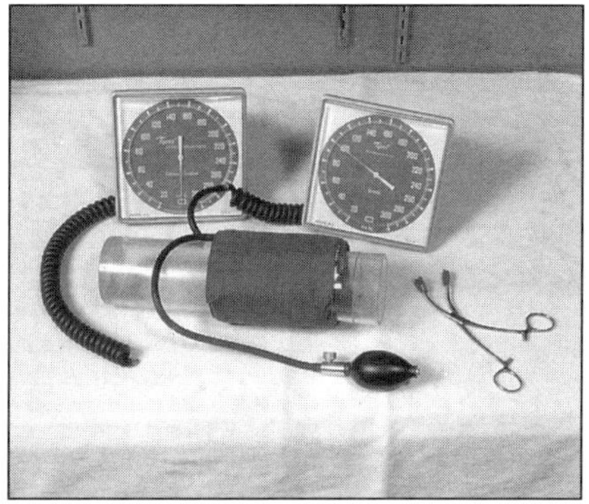

Figure 4-8 Both gauges should read the same pressure ± 5 mm Hg.

Result Sheet: Evacuated Tubes

Quality Control on Evacuated Blood Collection Tubes*

Date____________________ Lot No. ____________________

Tube size____________________ Tube color____________________

Expiration date____________ Checked by____________________

Each time a new lot number of tubes is placed into use, tubes must be checked as indicated below. Please sign off after checking the new lot number.

	Result
Visual inspection for anticoagulants	
Sterility of tube (if indicated)	
Check for clots by straining anticoagulated blood through gauze	
Sample spin-down	
Stopper pull-off	
Breakage from: Spinning	
Taking cap off	

*Adapted with permission. Garza D, Becan-McBride K. *Phlebotomy Handbook*. East Norwalk, Conn: Appleton and Lange; 1989:234.

Result Sheet: Needles

Date ____________________ Lot No. ____________________

Expiration date ________________________________

Needle gauge ____________________ Needle length ____________________

Result Sheet:
Centrifuges

Timing device

Setting 1	Reads__________	Timer__________
Setting 2	Reads__________	Timer__________
Setting 3	Reads__________	Timer__________

Tachometer reading:____________________

Acceptable range:____________________

Does the tachometer reading fall within an acceptable range for your model centrifuge?____________________

Result Sheet:
Blood Pressure Cuff

1. Does the aneroid gauge read "0" in the absence of pressure?__________

What is the appropriate course of action?____________________

____

2. Are there significant leaks in the tubing, inflating system, or exhaust valve?

____

____

3. Accuracy check/gauge. Pressure reading of original gauge:__________

Pressure reading of calibrated gauge:____________________

Do the readings vary by a significant difference?____________________

Based on the reading of the calibrated gauge, what is the appropriate course of action?____________________

Study Questions
Lab 4

1. List at least 5 tests that require a patient to be fasting prior to collection:

____

____

____

2. Define the following terms:

Aneroid: ______________________________

Petri dish: ______________________________

EDTA: ______________________________

National Bureau of Standards: ______________________________

National Committee for Clinical Laboratory Standards: ______________________________

____

3. How often are the following quality control procedures performed at your facility?

Accuracy check on the timing device for each centrifuge: ______________________________

Measurement of the RPMs on each centrifuge using a tachometer: ______________________________

____

Assessment of the inflating system of each blood pressure cuff: ______________________________

____

Assessment of the aneroid gauge for accuracy: ______________________________

____

LAB 5

Determining Total Volumes of Evacuated Tubes

Objective

To properly assemble the evacuated tube system; to learn how to determine the volume capacity of evacuated tubes; to evaluate evacuated tube fill volumes to determine whether or not the evacuated tube is filling to an acceptable level

Equipment

10 evacuated tubes with the following stopper colors:
Red (2 sizes), SST, Lavender (2 sizes), Blue (2 sizes), Gray, Green, Yellow;
1 standard-size holder; 1 small (pediatric) holder; 2 multidraw needles;
1 beaker of water; 1 graduated cylinder

Discussion

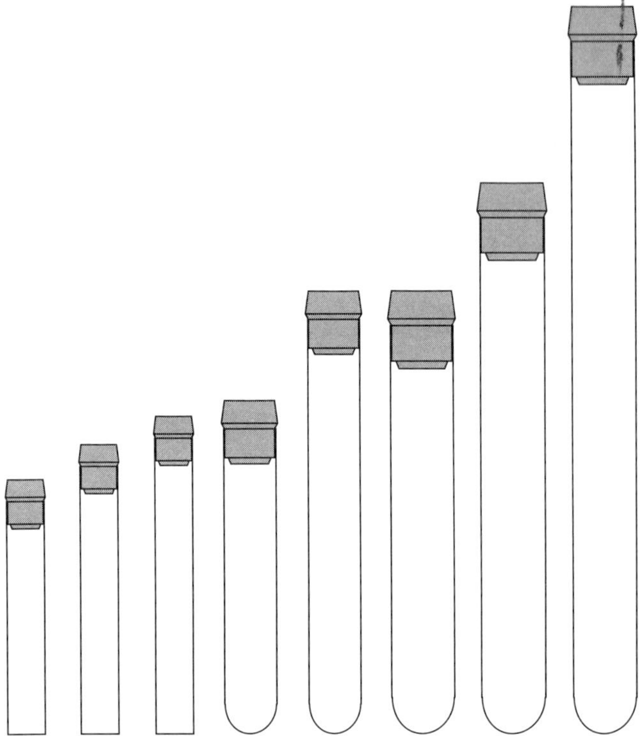

Figure 5-1 Examples of standard evacuated tube volumes.

In the previous lab, several pieces of equipment were evaluated to ensure quality specimen collection and/or quality test results. One aspect not detailed in the previous lab was acceptable volume filling of evacuated tubes.

The volume in an evacuated tube is calibrated to withdraw a particular amount of blood from a patient's vein. Evacuated tubes are manufactured in a variety of volume capacities, including, but not limited to, the following volumes: 2 mL, 3 mL, 4 mL, 5 mL, 7 mL, 10 mL, 15 mL, and 20 mL (**Fig. 5-1**).

Certain evacuated tubes contain additives. The evacuated tubes are manufactured to draw a volume of blood to react with the tube additive in a very specific blood:additive ratio. If the tube does not collect the appropriate amount of blood, the blood:additive ratio will be altered, which may impact the results of laboratory analysis performed in that specimen.

Evacuated tubes are manufactured with a variety of colored stoppers. The stopper color indicates which additive is inside the evacuated tube. Some evacuated tubes are typically used by certain departments. For example, hematology studies are often performed on specimens collected in EDTA tubes. Other evacuated tubes are typically used for particular tests. For example, specimens collected in sodium fluoride and thymol are used for glucose analysis only.

The following chart indicates the additives and properties of various evacuated tubes. (Note: The stopper colors in this workbook correspond to tubes manufactured by Becton Dickinson, Rutherford, New Jersey.)

Stopper Color	Additive	Anticoagulant	Mode of Action of Additive	Special Properties	Laboratory Department (Test Procedure)
Red	None	No	Not applicable	Used to collect specimens requiring serum and RBCs for analysis	Blood bank, Immunology
Red speckled or gold HEMOGARD	Serum separator gel	No	Serum: clot activator Separator gel: inert polymer gel acts as a barrier between serum and cells after centrifugation	Silica particles mix with the blood (during the inversion process) after collection to activate clot formation	Chemistry, RIA
Lavender	EDTA	Yes	Binds calcium	Prevents platelet clumping; prevents artifact formation on blood smears	Hematology
Blue	Sodium citrate	Yes	Binds calcium	Preserves labile factors; requires full draw	Coagulation
Green	Heparin	Yes	Neutralizes thrombin	Preserves structure of RBCs (anticoagulant of choice for osmotic fragility testing); is NOT used for blood smears stained with Wright's stain because the heparin reacts with the stain to form a blue background	Hematology (osmotic fragility, LE prep) Chemistry (pH, ammonia)
Gray	Potassium oxalate and sodium fluoride; or sodium fluoride and thymol	Yes	Precipitates calcium	Acts as a glycolytic inhibitor	Chemistry (glucose)
Yellow	Sodium polyanethole sulfonate (SPS)	Yes	Binds calcium	Acts as an anticoagulant; partially inactivates certain antibodies	Microbiology (blood cultures)
Navy (royal) 3 types	No additive Sodium heparin Sodium EDTA	Yes	None Neutralizes thrombin Binds calcium	Stoppers are manufactured without zinc stearate so that the specimen is not contaminated with zinc originating from the specimen stopper	Chemistry (trace metals such as zinc, copper, lead)

Volume Considerations

The effects of underfilling or overfilling evacuated tubes are listed in the chart below. The chart attempts to answer the question, "Is this amount of specimen sufficient for accurate analysis?" These volumes do NOT reflect volumes of blood consistent with quality control guidelines, but they are conservative estimates appropriate for most situations. It is difficult for a phlebotomist to accurately gauge the volume of blood collected in an evacuated tube at the patient's bedside. Therefore, conservative estimates of minimum acceptable volumes instead of actual minimum volumes are given as guidelines to ensure acceptable amounts of specimens.

Stopper Color	Overfill Effects	Underfill Effects	Minimum Acceptable Draw Volumes
Red	None	QNS	50% of capacity
Red speckled or gold HEMOGARD	There may not be sufficient clot activator for the entire specimen; centrifugation may be delayed waiting for complete clot formation to occur	QNS	50% of capacity
Lavender	Insufficient EDTA to completely inactivate clotting; results in clots within the specimen, rendering it inappropriate for testing	Dilution effect; erroneously low cell counts and hematocrits; RBC morphology changes; staining changes	50% of capacity
Blue	Insufficient sodium citrate to completely inactivate clotting; results in coagulation of the specimen, rendering it useless for testing	Prolongation of both PT and APTT results	100% of capacity
Green	Insufficient heparin to completely inactivate clotting; results in clotting of the specimen, rendering it useless for testing	Dilution effect; excess heparin may cause erroneously low results	50% of capacity
Gray	Insufficient additive to completely inactivate clotting; results in clotting of the specimen, rendering it useless for testing	Dilution effect; excess additive may cause erroneously low results	50% of capacity
Yellow	Insufficient SPS to completely inactivate clotting; results in bacteria trapped in clot and decreased bacterial counts	Decreased blood volume collection decreases the incidence of pathogen recovery	50% of capacity

The National Committee on Clinical Laboratory Standards (NCCLS) requires the actual draw to be ±10% of the labeled draw at the time of manufacture. For example, an evacuated tube scheduled to fill to a 10-mL capacity would have an acceptable fill range of 9 to 11 mL.

Calculation: 10 mL x .10 (10%) = 1 mL
10 – 1 = 9
10 + 1 = 11

Therefore, the acceptable fill range for an evacuated tube calibrated to fill to 10 mL is 9 to 11 mL.

Waste Disposal

Throughout this manual, attention will be given to the proper disposal of waste generated by the procedures performed. ANY needle, lancet, or syringe ("sharps" materials) used or opened during a laboratory procedure MUST be discarded in a needle disposal unit, which is made of thick plastic to prevent perforation by the contents (**Fig. 5-2**). Many needle disposal units have 2 kinds of openings in the top of the container. One opening is small and is intended to accommodate needles removed from evacuated tube holders or syringes. The second opening is larger and is designed to accommodate larger equipment, such as syringes, winged infusion needles, or partially filled evacuated tubes.

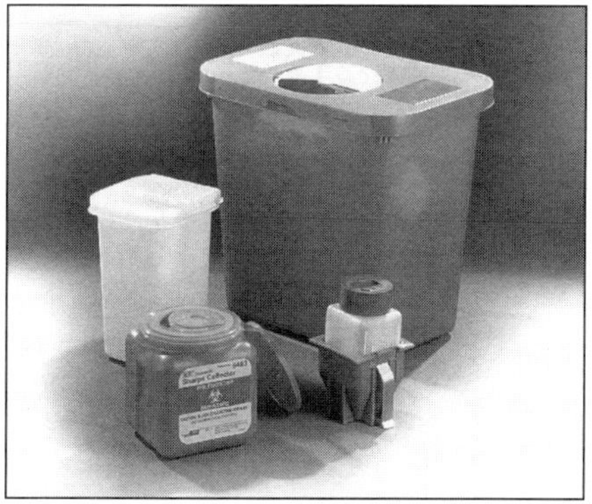

Figure 5-2 Examples of needle disposal units.

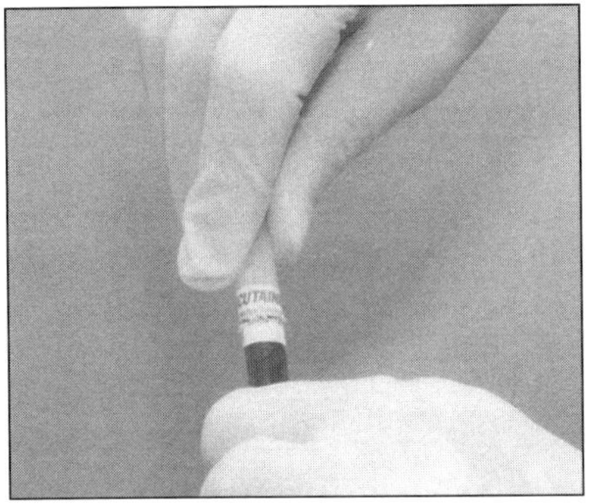

Figure 5-3 Twist cap of needle to break seal.

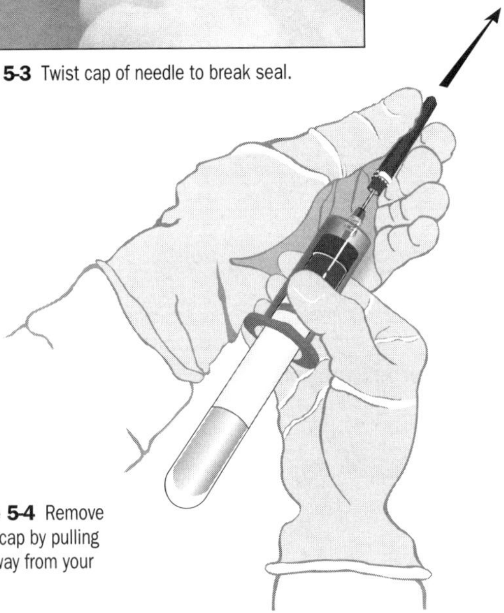

Figure 5-4 Remove needle cap by pulling it off away from your body.

Procedure 1: Filling Evacuated Tubes

1. Select, prepare, and organize the equipment. Obtain the equipment, as directed by your instructor. Open the needle by twisting off the protective paper seal or by snapping the protective plastic seal (**Fig. 5-3**). Secure the needle onto the standard-size holder. This is accomplished by screwing the needle firmly onto the holder. Keep your fingers on the outside of the holder while fastening the needle. NEVER touch either end of the needle. Place one of the larger evacuated tubes into the holder. The stopper should be against the needle, and the end of the tube should be outside of the holder. Arrange the remainder of the large-size evacuated tubes in the order the tubes will be loaded into the evacuated tube holder.
2. Remove the needle cover (**Fig. 5-4**) and submerge the bevel in the beaker of water.
3. Gently push down on the evacuated tube until the stopper is punctured by the back of the needle.
4. Continue to hold the bevel of the needle underneath the surface of the water until water stops entering the evacuated tube.
5. Keeping the bevel of the needle submerged, remove the first evacuated tube and replace it with the next one.
6. Continue filling and replacing evacuated tubes until all of the larger evacuated tubes have been filled.
7. Remove the last large evacuated tube from the holder.

8. Insert the needle into the appropriate opening in a needle disposal unit.
9. Fit the ridges located on the hub of the needle into the "teeth" of the opening of the needle disposal unit designed to accommodate needles (**Fig. 5-5**).
10. Detach the needle by unscrewing it from the holder (**Fig. 5-6**). Return holder to the original position and allow the needle to drop into the large opening (**Fig. 5-7**). NEVER use your fingers to push the needle into the disposal unit.
11. Prepare and organize the equipment listed for the small-size adapter. (Refer to step 1 above.)
12. Following the same procedure, fill the smaller-sized (pediatric) evacuated tubes.
13. After all of the smaller tubes have been filled, discard the needle into an appropriate needle disposal unit. (Refer to steps 8 through 10 above.)

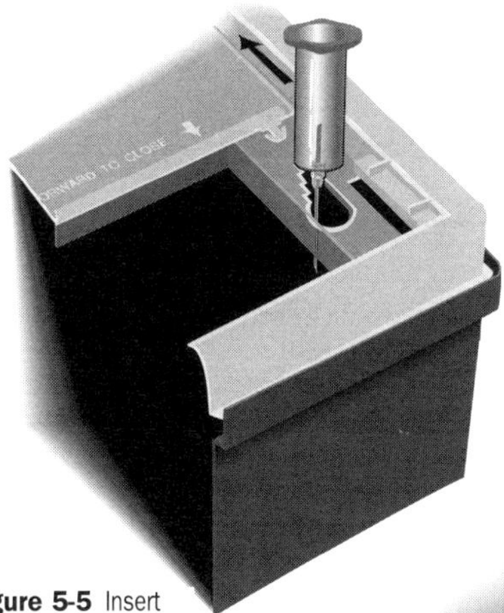

Figure 5-5 Insert needle into opening. Fit ridges on hub of needle into teeth in opening.

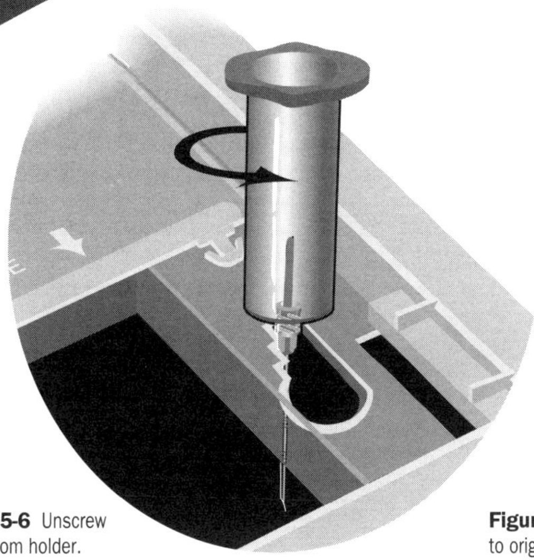

Figure 5-6 Unscrew needle from holder.

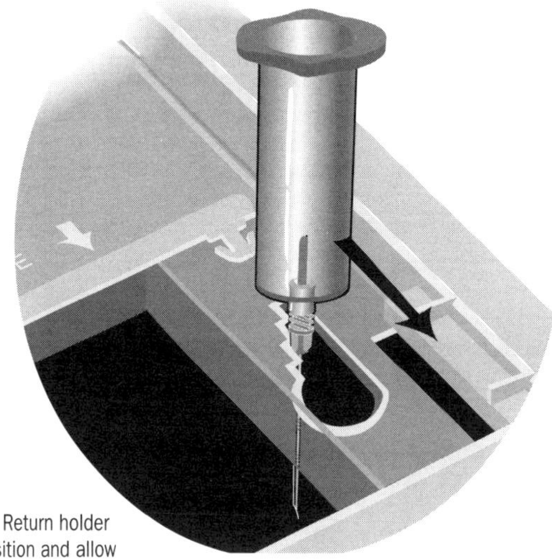

Figure 5-7 Return holder to original position and allow needle to drop into opening.

Procedure 2: Volume Measurement

1. Position the graduated cylinder on a flat surface.
2. Place a piece of gauze around the stopper of the first evacuated tube.
3. Remove the stopper by gently twisting it off.
4. Pour the water from the evacuated tube into the graduated cylinder.
5. To read a volume from a graduated cylinder, look at the marks (graduations) on the cylinder. For an accurate reading, the lines on the front of the cylinder must line up exactly with the lines on the back of the cylinder, from the observer's vantage point. The bottom of the meniscus corresponds to the volume of fluid in the graduated cylinder.
6. Record the volume on the result sheet.
7. Repeat steps 1 through 6 for each of the remaining evacuated tubes.
8. Complete the result sheet. For each evacuated tube, identify the following: 1) volume measured; 2) acceptable fill limits, as defined by NCCLS; 3) interpretation of the results, ie, determination of whether the volume measured falls within acceptable limits for quality volume draw; 4) additive; 5) laboratory department the test listed is performed in; 6) an example of a test for which each evacuated tube is used.

Result Sheet:

Determining Total Volumes of Evacuated Tubes

Stopper Color	Volume Measured	Acceptable Fill Limits (per NCCLS)	Interpretation A = Acceptable U = Unacceptable	Tube Additive	Example of a Test Collected in This Tube	Department Performing This Test	Comments
Red (Large)							
Red (Small)							
SST							
Lavender (Large)							
Lavender (Small)							
Blue (Large)							
Blue (Small)							
Gray							
Green							
Yellow							

Study Questions
Lab 5

1. Explain the difference between "binding calcium" and "precipitating calcium."
____

2. Define chelating: _______________

3. Write an example of a chemical formula that begins with an additive commonly used in evacuated tubes and that results in the precipitation of calcium: _____
____

4. Write an example of a chemical formula that begins with an additive commonly used in evacuated tubes and that results in the binding of calcium: _________
____

5. Define the following terms:

   Hemostasis: _______________

   Intrinsic pathway: _______________

   Extrinsic pathway: _______________

   Common pathway: _______________

   Fibrinolytic pathway: _______________

6. How do calcium and thrombin function in coagulation in vivo? _______________
____

7. How does inactivating calcium and thrombin in vitro result in preventing blood from clotting? _______________
____

LAB 6

Selection and Preparation of an Appropriate Site for Skin Puncture

Objective

To introduce and familiarize the student with appropriate sites for skin puncture; to introduce and familiarize the student with preparation of a site prior to skin puncture

Equipment

Doll; 2 70% isopropyl alcohol prep pads; Sterile gauze; Heel warmer; Blood lancet; Gown; Gloves

Patient Identification

Before the collection of ANY type of blood specimen, the patient must be properly identified. Quality laboratory analysis begins with proper patient identification. There is absolutely NO margin of error in the procedure of patient identification.

Blood tests are performed for a variety of reasons. Physicians' selection of a course of treatment for patients often depends on the results of laboratory analysis ordered to evaluate the patient's condition. If a blood specimen is collected from the wrong patient, the patient may receive inappropriate treatment with potentially disastrous consequences. For example, if a patient is incorrectly identified for type and crossmatch specimen collection, the patient may receive an incompatible unit of blood. This may result in the patient's death.

Proper patient identification is a 2-step identification procedure.

1 The first step in patient identification for both inpatients and outpatients is to ask the patient to state his/her first and last name. If the patient is unable to state his/her name, a family member or a member of the nursing staff may provide verbal identification.

2 The second—and most important—step in inpatient identification is to confirm patient identification information from the test requisition with the patient identification information found on the patient's wristband. The wristband must be attached to the patient. For example, wristbands taped to beds or hanging on cribs are unacceptable for use in patient identification. Identification information from the test requisition form must ALWAYS be confirmed with the patient's wristband before a blood specimen may be collected.

The second step in outpatient identification requires confirmation of personal information on the test requisition with the patient. For example, the phlebotomist may ask the patient to recite his/her address or social security number to ensure proper patient identification.

Site Selection/ Heelstick

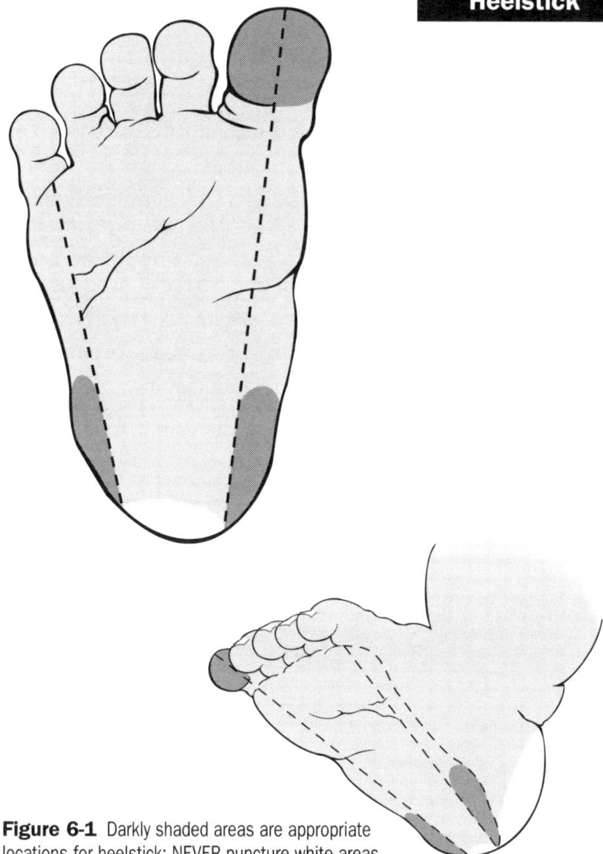

Figure 6-1 Darkly shaded areas are appropriate locations for heelstick; NEVER puncture white areas.

When performing skin punctures on infants, care must be exercised to perform the puncture in appropriate areas of the heel. Puncturing unacceptable areas can cause complications, including osteochondritis, sepsis, and gangrene.

The puncture should be made on the most lateral or medial portions of the plantar surface. Although the procedure for skin puncture in infants is commonly termed "heelstick," the puncture should NEVER be performed on the posterior curvature of the heel. Bones in the infant's foot are twice as close to the skin at the back of the foot than on the bottom or plantar surface of the foot.

The area encompassed by imaginary lines drawn between the heel and the big toe and the heel and the fourth toe is not appropriate for heelstick, because of the possibility of hitting bone, which could result in infection and osteomyelitis. The areas outside of this zone are the most appropriate locations (**Fig. 6-1**).

The puncture should NOT be performed: on the posterior curvature of the heel; on the arch area of the foot (puncture in this area may result in injury to nerves, cartilage, and tendons and offers no advantage over any other acceptable area of the foot); on an area with bruises or abrasions present; or through previous puncture sites.

Site Selection/ Fingerstick

Fingersticks should be performed on the palmar surface of the distal phalanx of the index, ring, or middle finger (**Fig. 6-2**). Middle or ring fingers are most desirable, since the index finger has an increased number of nerve endings and is therefore more sensitive. The sides and the tips of the distal phalanx should NOT be used, as the tissue on this area of the finger is only half as thick as that on the palmar surface. The fifth finger is not used for skin puncture, as the tissue on this finger is considerably thinner than that on other fingers. Fingersticks should be performed perpendicular to the fingerprints. If the puncture is made parallel to the fingerprints, the blood will channel down the patient's finger instead of forming a drop at the puncture site, making collection much more difficult.

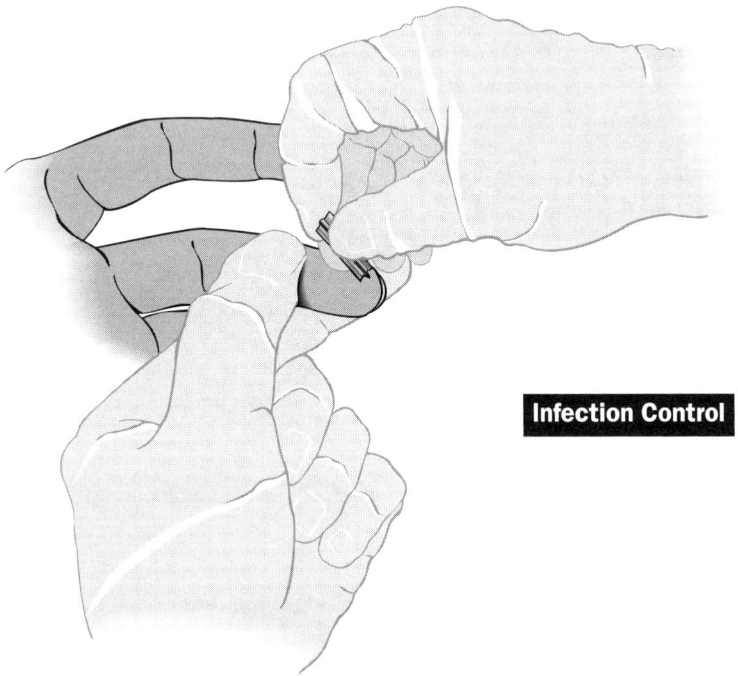

Figure 6-2 Appropriate technique for grasping finger for fingerstick.

Infection Control

Because babies have immature immune systems, some facilities require personnel to wear protective clothing into the nursery to prevent the spread of infection to the neonate. Most facilities require that health care workers entering the nursery wear gowns and gloves. Some facilities also require masks in the nursery.

Site Preparation

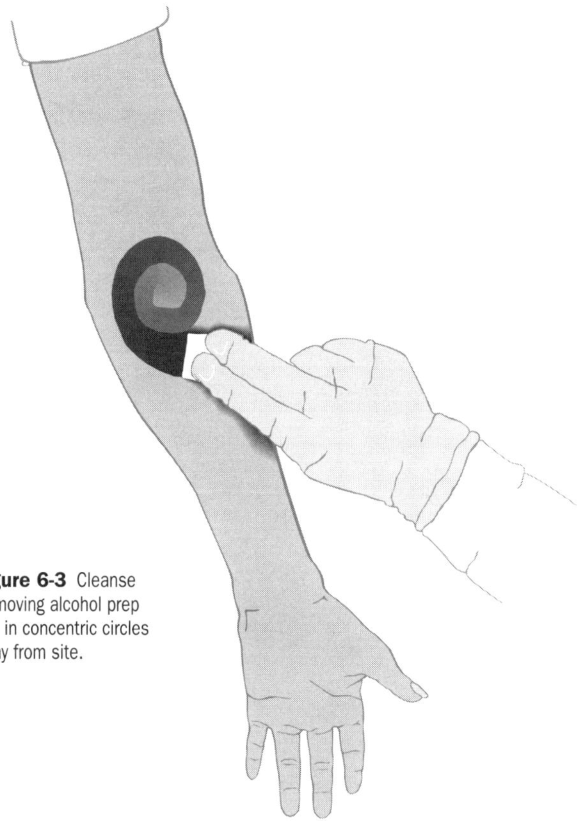

Figure 6-3 Cleanse by moving alcohol prep pad in concentric circles away from site.

Although variable from person to person, many bacteria are present on the skin. Introduction of bacteria on the skin surface into the puncture site may result in an infected site. Therefore, prior to performing a skin puncture, the site must be decontaminated. Decontamination is accomplished by applying 70% isopropyl alcohol to the puncture site. Variations in application technique exist in the field. Some facilities instruct personnel to rub the site vigorously with the alcohol pad. Other facilities instruct personnel to apply the alcohol prep pad to the puncture site and cleanse the site by moving the alcohol prep pad in concentric circles away from the puncture site (**Fig. 6-3**). This workbook will provide instruction in the latter technique.

Applying heat to the skin puncture site can significantly increase blood flow to the site. There are 2 methods of warming a skin puncture site.

1. A towel moistened in warm (39–42°C) water is used to cover the site for a period of 3 minutes. The temperature of the water moistening the towel must not exceed 42°C. Water temperatures exceeding 42°C can burn an infant's skin.

2. A commercially prepared warmer may be applied to the selected skin puncture site. The warmer contains the components of a heat-generating chemical reaction. The reaction is initiated by either squeezing the unit to mix the chemicals or by bending back and forth a metal disk contained within the unit. (The exact procedure is determined by the type of warmer purchased by the facility.) This triggers a chemical reaction that produces heat for approximately 5 minutes.

Procedure 1: Heelstick Preparation

(following nursery technique, to be performed on the doll)

1. Wash hands.
2. Don gown and gloves.
3. Role play: Identify the patient, using the 2-step method of patient identification. (A fellow student may act as the infant's parents or a member of the nursing staff.)
4. Warm the selected site, using heel warmer.
5. Select, prepare, and organize equipment. Obtain the necessary equipment, as directed by your instructor. Open the alcohol prep pad package. Do NOT remove the alcohol pad! Open the lancet packaging. Peel the packaging apart, following the directions of your instructor. Do NOT remove the lancet from the packaging! If the lancet and alcohol are removed from their respective packaging and placed on a nonsterile surface, they may become contaminated. Arrange the equipment in the order it will be used during the procedure. The equipment should be arranged in a location that will make it easily accessible during the procedure.
6. Select area for puncture site.
7. Remove alcohol prep pad from package.
8. Grasp the infant's foot in the following manner: place the forefinger over the arch of the foot; place the thumb below the puncture site; place the remaining 3 fingers on top of the foot, in front of the shin bone (**Fig. 6-4**).
9. Clean the site, beginning at the puncture site, and move the pad in concentric circles outward.
10. Allow the site to air dry.
11. Apply the BLUNT end of the lancet on the site selected and cleaned to indicate the position of the puncture.

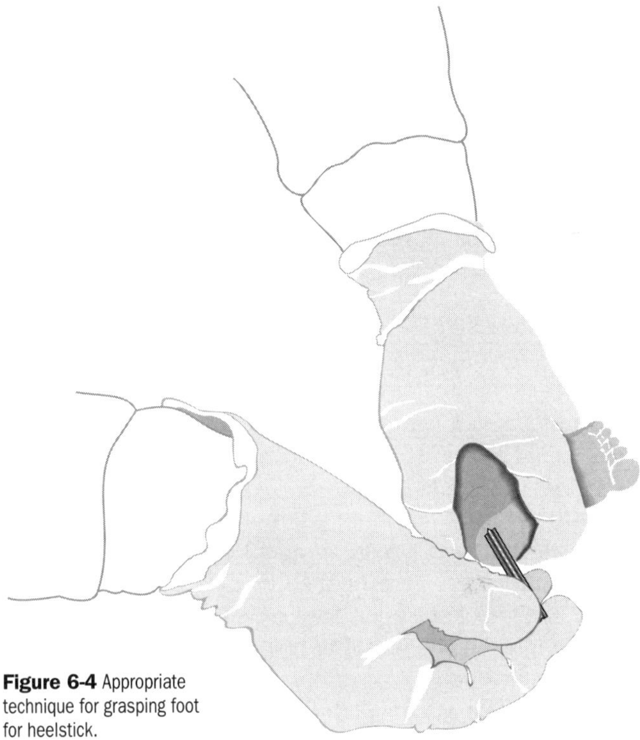

Figure 6-4 Appropriate technique for grasping foot for heelstick.

Procedure 2: Fingerstick Preparation

(to be performed on your lab partner)

1. Wash hands. Don gloves and gown.
2. Role play: Identify patient, using the 2-step method of patient identification.
3. Select, prepare, and organize equipment (refer to Procedure 1, step 5).
4. Select site for skin puncture.
5. Gently massage finger chosen, from hand to fingertip, 3 to 4 times.
6. If the patient's hand is cold, apply a heel warmer to the skin puncture site.
7. Remove alcohol prep pad from package.
8. Clean the site, using a circular motion, beginning at the puncture site and moving outward.
9. Allow the area to air dry.
10. Apply the blunt end of the lancet to the puncture site, perpendicular to the fingerprints, to indicate the position of the puncture (**Fig. 6-5**).

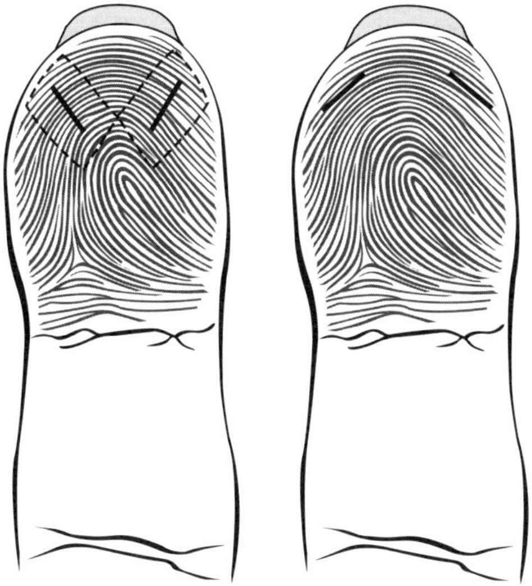

Figure 6-5 Left, appropriate location for lancet placement for fingerstick; right, inappropriate location for lancet placement.

Assignment

Practice both procedures at least 3 times. Once competency has been achieved in both procedures to the satisfaction of your lab partner, perform both procedures for your instructor. Your competency will be assessed by the instructor using the following checklist.

Checklist:

Skin Puncture

(A) Performed **(B) Needs Improvement** **(C) Not Performed**

Comments:

_____1. Washes hands before starting the procedure.
_____2. Dons gloves and gown.
_____3. Selects, prepares, and organizes equipment.
_____4. Identifies patient, using 2-step method of patient identification.
_____5. Selects site for skin puncture.
_____6. Applies warmer to site when appropriate.
_____7. Cleanses skin puncture site with alcohol.
_____8. Allows site to air dry.
_____9. Secures puncture site appropriately.
_____10. Applies blunt end of lancet to the puncture site at an appropriate angle.
_____11. Applies blunt end of lancet to an appropriate site for skin puncture.
_____12. Discards lancet in needle disposal unit.

Study Questions
Lab 6

Please note: While it is ONLY appropriate for physicians to diagnose conditions and treat patients, it is important for students to realize the meaning of potential complications of inappropriately performed skin punctures. Questions 1 through 6 are included to assist the student in researching the exact meaning of the terms used to describe potential complications of inappropriately performed skin puncture and the commonly prescribed treatment of each complication.

1. List at least 3 symptoms of osteochondritis: ______________________________

____

____

____

2. How is osteochondritis commonly treated? ______________________________

____

3. List at least 3 symptoms of gangrene: ______________________________

____

____

4. How is gangrene commonly treated? ______________________________

____

5. List at least 3 symptoms of sepsis: ______________________________

____

____

6. How is sepsis commonly treated? ______________________________

____

7. Define basal state: ______________________________

____

8. If a patient is NOT in the basal state when blood is collected, the laboratory results may be affected. List at least 6 changes in the patient's physical disposition that may affect laboratory results:

____

____

____

____

____

____

LAB 7

Introduction to Venipuncture Site Selection

Objective

To introduce and familiarize the student with appropriate sites for routine venipuncture; to introduce and familiarize the student with preparation of a site prior to venipuncture

Equipment

Tourniquet;
70% isopropyl alcohol prep pads

Positioning of the Tourniquet

The tourniquet should be positioned approximately 3 to 4 inches above the area to be examined as a potential venipuncture site (**Fig. 7-1**). If a patient's arm is particularly hairy, has a skin disorder, or is particularly sensitive to the tourniquet, the tourniquet may be placed over the patient's sleeve.

The tourniquet is applied to increase venous filling. This makes the veins more pronounced and easier to access. The tourniquet should never be left on for longer than 1 minute. If a tourniquet is left on for longer than 1 minute, certain test results may be affected because localized stasis (ie, stoppage of blood flow) may occur. A partial filtrate of the blood will be formed, and hemoconcentration will occur. These circumstances may result in falsely elevated levels for all protein-based analytes (eg, enzymes), hematocrit levels, and other cellular levels.

Applying the Tourniquet

Cross the ends in front of the patient's arm (**Fig. 7-2**). Hold one end of the tourniquet in each hand. Pull one end tight (**Fig. 7-3**) and grasp the intersection

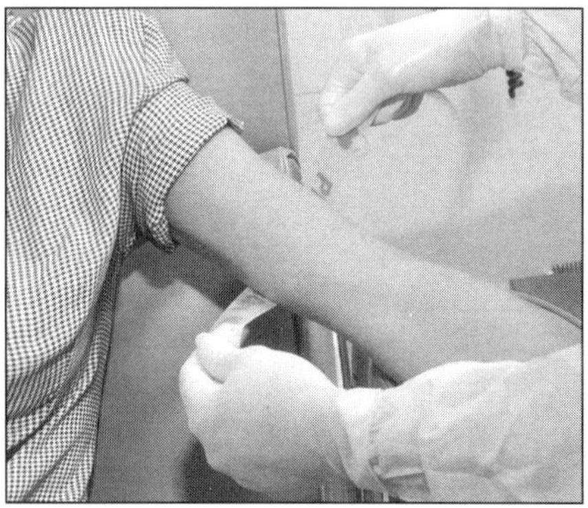

Figure 7-1 Appropriate location for tourniquet.

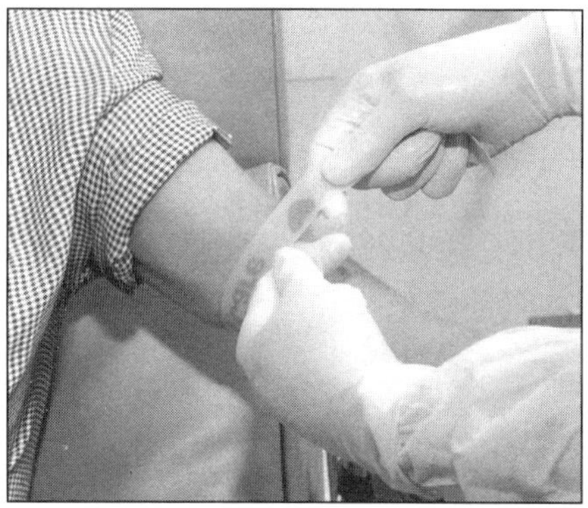

Figure 7-2 Cross ends in front of patient's arm.

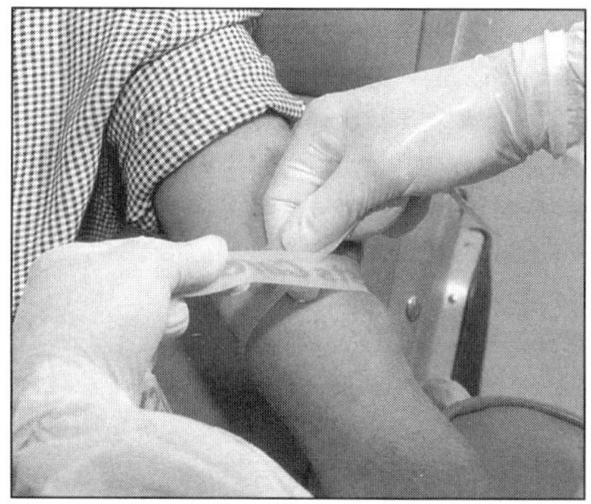

Figure 7-3 Pull one end tight.

between the thumb and forefinger of one hand (**Fig. 7-4**). Tuck the portion of the tourniquet closed to and positioned on the bottom of the intersection into the top of the intersection to form a loop with the end pointing toward the upper part of the patient's body (**Fig. 7-5**, **Fig. 7-6**, **Fig. 7-7**).

If the tourniquet is too loose, it will slip off the patient's arm. Another indication of a tourniquet tied too loosely is failure of the veins to become turgid (ie, full or distended). If the tourniquet is too loose, the appropriate course of action is to release it and retie it, pulling the ends tighter so the intersection of the ends occurs closer to the patient's arm.

Indications of a tourniquet applied too tightly include: white color of the patient's skin in the area of the tied tourniquet; appearance of petechiae (ie, small, pinpoint bruises) on the patient's arm; reddish purple coloring of the patient's hand; or a complaint by the patient.

If the tourniquet is applied too tightly, the appropriate course of action is to untie the tourniquet and retie it. Position the ends of the tourniquet so the intersection is positioned further away from the patient's arm.

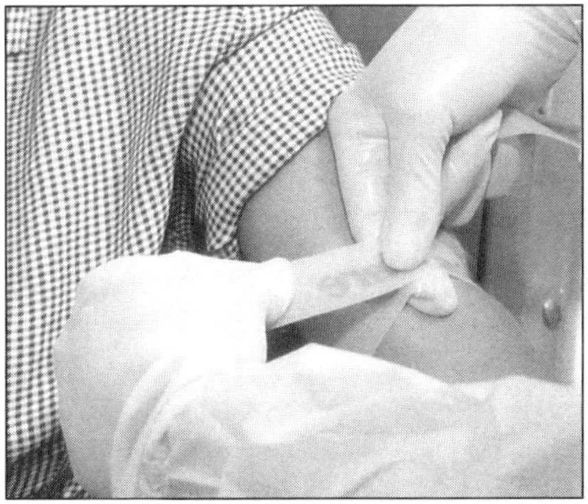

Figure 7-4 Grasp the intersection of the tourniquet.

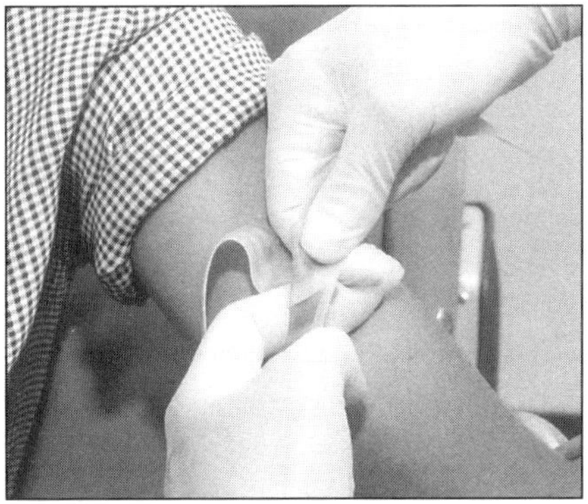

Figure 7-5 Tuck the bottom end in to form a loop.

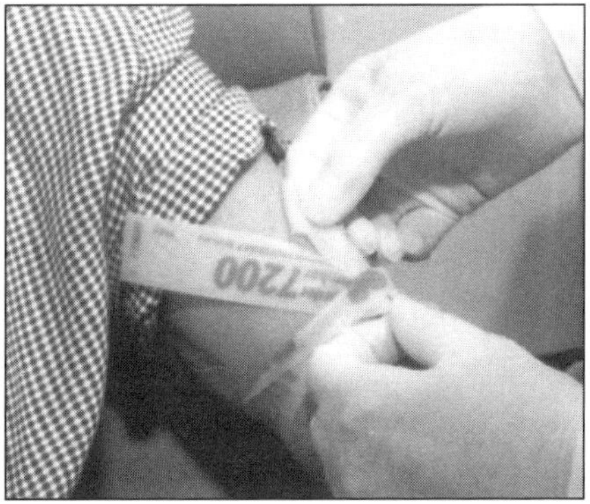

Figure 7-6 Pull the loop through the bottom.

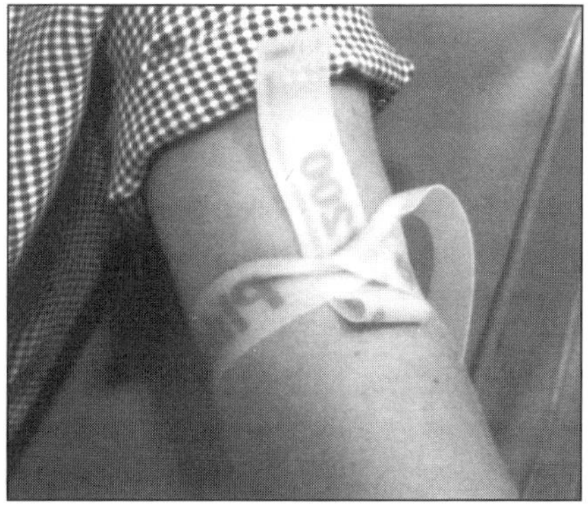

Figure 7-7 Appropriately tied tourniquet.

Site Selection

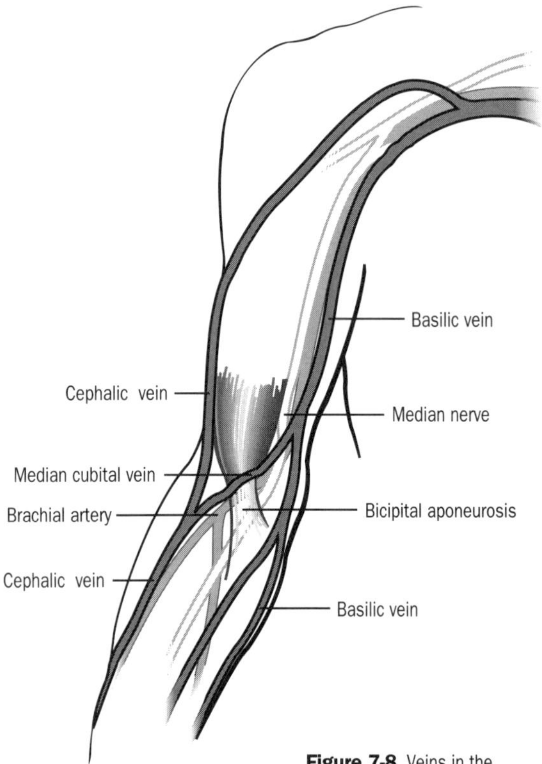

Figure 7-8 Veins in the antecubital fossa.

Choosing an appropriate site for venipuncture is crucial to the success of the procedure. Veins most often considered for use during venipuncture include the median cubital vein (venae mediana cubiti), cephalic vein (venae cephalica), and basilic vein (venae basilica) (**Fig. 7-8**). The order of vein selection for venipuncture is as follows: 1) median cubital vein; 2) cephalic vein; and 3) basilic vein.

The median cubital vein is the first choice because it is usually one of the largest, fullest veins in the antecubital area of the arm (the area in front of the elbow). It is also the vein that is best anchored by the surrounding musculature, which makes it easier to access by venipuncture. The cephalic vein is also a large, full vein appearing on the "thumb side" of the antecubital area of the arm. It is not as well anchored by surrounding musculature as the median cubital vein, but it is better anchored than the basilic vein. The basilic vein is generally smaller than either the median cubital or cephalic veins. It is also not particularly well anchored by surrounding musculature. Consequently, the phlebotomist must exercise particular caution to ensure that the basilic vein is anchored well before making the venipuncture. Improper or inadequate anchoring of the basilic vein may cause it to "roll" away from the needle, requiring a readjustment of the needle or a second venipuncture. Both of these circumstances will cause additional pain to the patient.

If a patient has more than one vein in the antecubital area suitable for venipuncture, the phlebotomist must choose which one is most likely to ensure a successful venipuncture. Most phlebotomists select the largest vein. If the veins are comparable in size, the order of selection is as follows: median cubital vein, cephalic vein, and basilic vein.

The median cubital vein is best anchored in the surrounding musculature. Therefore, it is less likely to move, or "roll," when the phlebotomist attempts to insert the needle. The cephalic vein has some support from surrounding musculature, but not as much as the median cubital vein. The basilic vein is often not well anchored by surrounding musculature, which makes it more difficult to access. In addition, the basilic vein is located close to the brachial artery, introducing an

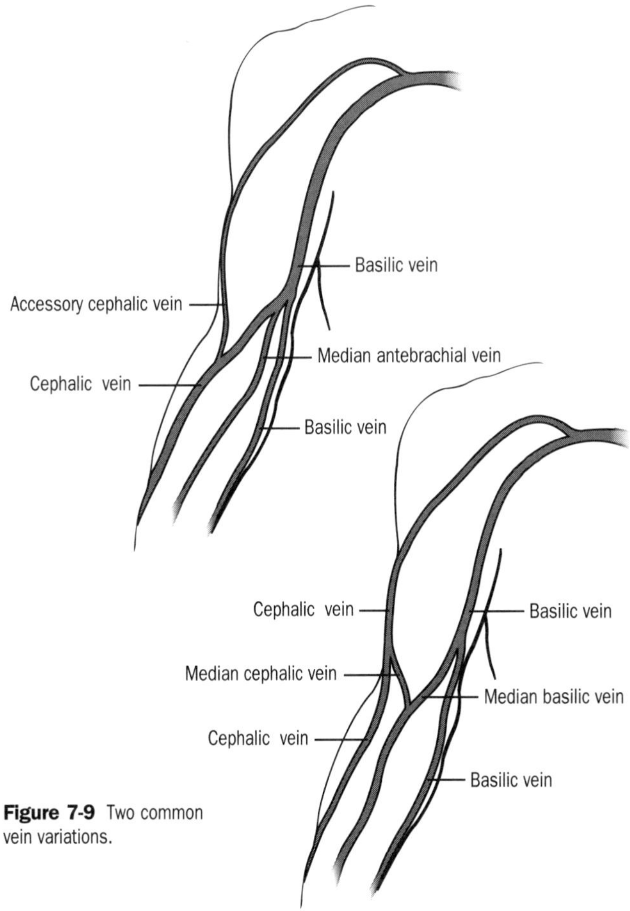

Figure 7-9 Two common vein variations.

additional hazard of accidental arterial puncture. Finally, the section of the antecubital area in which the basilic vein is located seems to be more sensitive, so that venipuncture in this area of the arm is more painful to the patient. The phlebotomist should always assess a vein's tendency to move or "roll" when evaluating it as a possible venipuncture site.

Most patients do not have veins as diagrammed in **Figure 7-8**. In fact, most of the time the phlebotomist does not have a choice between several veins. Most often, phlebotomists are relieved if a patient has 1 vein suitable for venipuncture in a single antecubital area. Two examples of variations in vein structure are shown in **Figure 7-9**.

To select a vein suitable for venipuncture, palpate the antecubital area with your index finger. Gently but firmly push down on the skin. If you are palpating a vein, you will be able to feel the vein bounce back when you lift your finger from the site. (Push down with your finger and release until you locate a structure that feels similar to a stretched rubber band underneath the skin.) In addition to location, the vein should be assessed to determine the width, depth, and direction of the vein. Vein selection is based on the location and size of the vein. The largest naturally anchored vein should be the phlebotomist's first choice.

The phlebotomist should assess the vein to determine where its structure is deepest and widest and in what direction it is situated in the patient's arm. The needle should be inserted in the widest, deepest part of the vein and in the same direction as the vein.

Procedure

Venipuncture Site Selection

1. Apply the tourniquet.
2. Palpate the antecubital fossa, using the index finger.
3. Identify the blood vessels in the patient's arm.
4. Select the BEST site for venipuncture.
5. Untie the tourniquet.
6. Cleanse the venipuncture site selected, using the alcohol prep pad. Beginning at the puncture site, move the alcohol pad in concentric circles outward.
7. Retie the tourniquet. Be careful not to touch the venipuncture site with the tourniquet.

Assignment

Repeat the procedure on at least 3 different persons. Once competency has been achieved, to your satisfaction, perform the procedure for your instructor. Your competency will be assessed by the instructor using the following checklist.

Checklist:

Venipuncture Site Selection

Comments:

(A) Performed **(B) Needs Improvement** **(C) Not Performed**

______1. Positions tourniquet so it is tied 3 to 4 inches above the antecubital fossa.
______2. Positions tourniquet over clothing, if appropriate.
______3. Appropriately ties tourniquet.
______4. Ties tourniquet neither too loose nor too tight.
______5. Palpates antecubital fossa with index finger.
______6. Identifies the veins present in the patient's arm.
______7. Identifies the most suitable vein for venipuncture.
______8. Provides appropriate rationale for vein selected.
______9. Determines size and direction of each vein identified.
______10. Selects most appropriate site for venipuncture.
______11. Unties tourniquet within 1 minute.
______12. Appropriately unties tourniquet.
______13. Cleanses site, using concentric circular motion.
______14. Reties tourniquet without touching selected venipuncture site.

Study Questions
Lab 7

1. What is the most important step in a venipuncture procedure?

2. What is the difference between whole blood, serum, and plasma?

3. When is the appropriate time for a blood specimen to be labeled?

4. A patient has an IV line running in the right arm and a full cast on the left arm. What are some alternative sites for blood draw?

5. After tying the tourniquet on a patient's arm, the phlebotomist palpates the antecubital area. An artery, 2 veins, and a tendon are palpated. How can the phlebotomist tell the difference between each structure, using the sense of touch?

6. How should blood be mixed with additives in evacuated tubes?

7. When should the mixing take place?

LAB 8
The Duke Bleeding Time

Objective

To introduce the following skills: patient communication, including patient approach and patient identification; skin puncture procedures, including site preparation and skin puncture, using a blood lancet; timing procedures for bleeding times, as an introduction to the modified Ivy template bleeding time; and disposal of waste materials, especially the disposal of biohazardous waste

Equipment

Gloves; Gown; 70% isopropyl alcohol prep pad; Filter paper; Stopwatch; 3-mm sterile lancet; Needle disposal unit; Biohazard bag

Discussion

The Duke bleeding time involves performing a skin puncture on a patient's earlobe and determining the time it takes for the wound to stop bleeding. Even though the Duke bleeding time is an outdated procedure, it is incorporated into this laboratory workbook as a teaching tool.

The Duke bleeding time is an effective introductory procedure for phlebotomy students, offering the following advantages:

- The Duke bleeding time allows the student to practice several patient interaction techniques, including patient approach, patient identification, and patient interview concerning patient preparation for the procedure.
- The Duke bleeding time is a relatively painless procedure, thereby allowing students to perform an initial phlebotomy procedure on a fellow student without causing much pain.
- The Duke bleeding time allows the student acting as patient to be introduced to the role of a patient being subjected to a phlebotomy procedure, while keeping specimen volume to a minimum.
- The Duke bleeding time usually does not generate a large volume of specimen, which introduces the student to procedures involving biohazardous materials on a small scale. The student may become acclimated to working with blood, gloves, and disposal of biohazardous materials without the additional anxiety of dealing with a large volume of sample.
- The Duke bleeding time introduces the student to the concept of timing a procedure, which is a basic skill to be reintroduced later in the modified Ivy template bleeding time procedure.

The Duke bleeding time, named for the person who developed the procedure, was originally described in 1910. The variability of earlobe thickness and puncture depth results in poor reproducibility and, therefore, unreliable results. Consequently, in current clinical practice, the Duke bleeding time is being performed less frequently in deference to the more standardized modified Ivy bleeding time.

Clinical Significance

Bleeding time is an assay used to assess the contributions of platelet function and blood vessel integrity to primary blood-clotting abilities. It is widely utilized as a presurgical screening tool to detect disorders of primary hemostasis, such as von Willebrand's disease, congenital or acquired platelet defects, and vascular disorders. Various physiologic factors, such as platelet count, platelet function, circulating von Willebrand factor, and vascular tone, can influence test results.

Aspirin and aspirin-containing compounds affect platelet functioning and consequently may affect the results of the bleeding time test. Aspirin may affect platelet functioning for as long as 7 to 10 days.

Patient Approach

According to "A Patient's Bill of Rights," approved by the House of Delegates of the American Hospital Association on February 6, 1973, a patient has the right to certain information when approached by a health care worker. The patient has the right to know the health care worker's name, the department the health care worker represents, and the reason the health care worker is approaching the patient. If, during the interview, the patient asks the phlebotomist for information concerning the nature of the tests the physician has ordered, the phlebotomist should always refer the patient to the physician for information. The physician orders tests and evaluates the results within the context of each patient's condition. The phlebotomist is not trained to provide this sort of information. It is the physician's responsibility to discuss the laboratory tests ordered and the results with the patient.

Prior to performing a procedure, health care workers may introduce themselves as follows: "Hello, my name is (state your name). I am from the laboratory, and I'm here to perform a test that your doctor has ordered."

After identifying themselves, phlebotomists should appropriately identify the patient (refer to Lab #6). Following patient identification, the phlebotomist should explain the procedure to be performed. For example, "Your doctor has requested a test that is performed on your earlobe. It involves briefly puncturing the earlobe with a lancet. I will measure how long it takes for the bleeding to stop. Do you have any questions?" The phlebotomist may respond to any questions the patient has concerning the procedure ONLY. If the patient inquires about the significance of the test relative to his/her condition, he/she should be referred to the physician who ordered the test. The patient then should be questioned concerning prescription and over-the-counter medications taken during the previous 7 to 10 days. If the patient has taken aspirin or aspirin-containing compounds during the previous 7 to 10 days, a supervisor should be notified before continuing with the procedure (see list below). If a patient questions a phlebotomist concerning a particular test, the appropriate course of action for the phlebotomist is to refer the patient to the physician. The patient's physician can interpret test results within the context of each patient's condition.

Common Drugs Containing Aspirin

- Alka-Seltzer
- Anacin
- Anahist
- APC
- APC with codeine
- APC with demerol
- ASA
- ASA compound
- ASA compound with codeine
- Aspergum
- Aspirin (USP)
- Aspirin, children's
- Bayer
- Bayer, children's
- Bayer timed-release
- Bufferin
- Calurin
- Cama inlay
- Cope
- Coricidin
- Coricidin "D"
- Coricidin demilets
- Coricidin medilets
- Darvon with ASA
- Darvon-N with ASA
- Darvon Compound
- Dolene
- Dristan
- Ecotrin
- Empiral
- Empirin
- Empirin with codeine
- Emprazil
- Emprazil-C
- Equagesic
- Excedrin
- Excedrin PM
- Fiorinal
- Fiorinal with codeine
- Fizrin
- Four-way cold tablets
- Liquiprin
- Measurin
- Midol
- Norgesic
- PAC compound
- PAC compound with codeine
- Percodan
- Robaxisal
- Robaxisal-pH
- Sine-off
- St. Joseph
- St. Joseph for children
- Super-anahist
- Synalgos
- Synalgos-DC
- Triaminicin
- Vanquish

Sources of Error

Errors in the performance of the Duke bleeding time may be caused by the phlebotomist, the equipment, or the procedure itself.

Patient identification: Quality results always begin with proper patient identification. Positive identification of the patient before performing any procedure is the phlebotomist's chief responsibility.

Patient interview: If the patient has taken aspirin or aspirin-containing compounds 7 to 10 days prior to the procedure, the bleeding time may be prolonged. The phlebotomist must determine the patient's history concerning aspirin ingestion to ensure quality results.

Improper puncture: Results may be affected by an improperly performed puncture. A puncture that is too shallow, too deep, or in an inappropriate location will adversely affect test results.

Alcohol: The alcohol must be completely dried before making the puncture. If residual alcohol is on a puncture site, the bleeding time will be erroneously prolonged.

Timing: If the phlebotomist does not initiate timing of the procedure simultaneously with the puncture, the results will be adversely affected.

Filter paper: If the phlebotomist allows the filter paper to touch the wound, the platelet clot may be dislodged, causing falsely elevated results.

Stopwatch: If the stopwatch has not been appropriately calibrated, it may keep incorrect time. Stopwatches should be calibrated on a regular basis as a part of the quality assurance program.

Standardization: The procedural source of error for the Duke bleeding time is the inability to standardize the puncture. This error is considerable, since it prevents reproducibility, and therefore reliability of results. For this reason, most facilities have substituted a modified Ivy bleeding time procedure for the Duke bleeding time.

Procedure 1: Duke Bleeding Time

1. Wash hands. Don gloves and gown.
2. Role play: Approach the patient. Introduce yourself and the department you represent. Indicate that you will be performing a test that the patient's physician has ordered. Ask the patient if he/she has taken any aspirin or aspirin-containing medications within the last 7 to 10 days. If the patient is wearing pierced earrings, request that they be removed from the ear for the procedure.
3. Role play: Identify the patient, using the 2-step method of patient identification.
4. Role play: Explain the procedure to the patient. Do NOT offer information related to the clinical significance of the procedure! Remember, information concerning rationale for test procedures is the domain of the physician.
5. Select, prepare, and organize equipment. Assemble the equipment listed above. Peel back the package of the lancet. Do NOT remove the lancet from the packaging. Position the opened package so the lancet may be removed easily from the packaging during the procedure. Open the alcohol prep pad. Position the equipment in order of use during the procedure. Read the procedure before performing the Duke bleeding time to determine the order the equipment is used.
6. Remove the alcohol prep pad from the packaging. Unfold the alcohol prep pad. Place one half of the prep pad in front of the earlobe, and the second half behind the earlobe.
7. Cleanse the patient's earlobe by moving the prep pad back and forth along the earlobe.
8. Allow the site to air dry.

9. Grasp the patient's earlobe between your thumb and index finger (**Fig. 8-1**).
10. Using the sterile lancet, make a puncture at the base of the earlobe (**Fig. 8-2**). Simultaneously start the stopwatch.
11. Blot (wick) the blood with filter paper (without touching the wound) every 30 seconds, until the bleeding has stopped (**Fig. 8-3**). Touching the wound with the filter paper will dislodge the platelet plug formed during primary hemostasis, falsely increasing the bleeding time.
12. When the blood no longer stains the filter paper, stop the timer. Record the time to the nearest 30 seconds.
13. Dispose of refuse in the following manner: used lancets in the needle disposal unit; blood-contaminated items in a biohazard bag; and noncontaminated items (lancet packaging, alcohol prep, etc) in the appropriate trash receptacle.

Normal values: 1 to 3 minutes; borderline values: 3 to 6 minutes

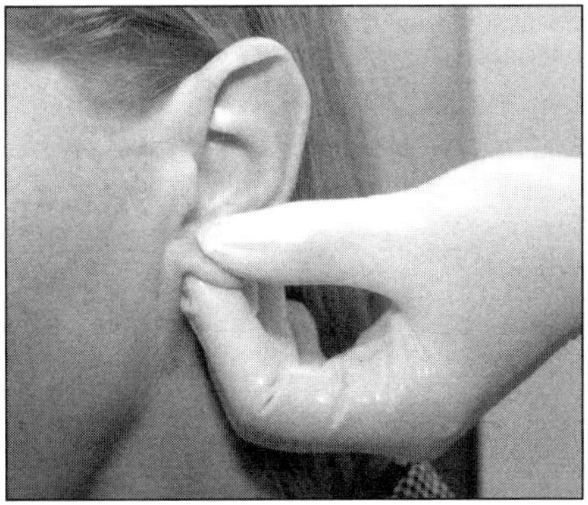

Figure 8-1 Grasp the earlobe.

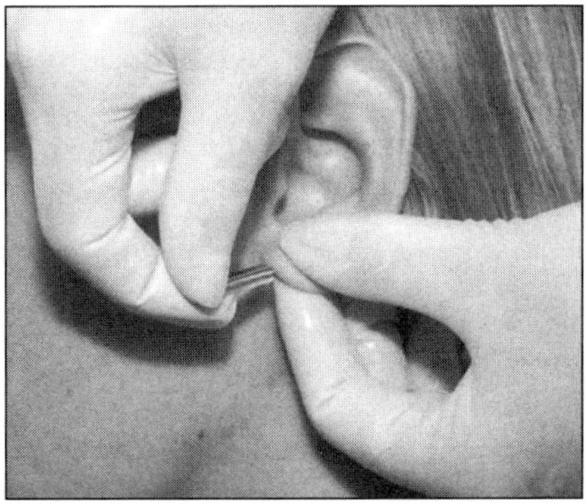

Figure 8-2 Puncture base of earlobe with lancet.

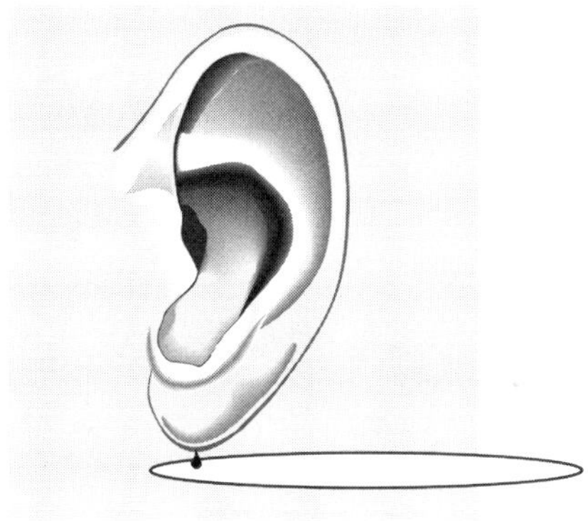

Figure 8-3 Wick the blood without touching the wound.

Procedure 2: Unsuccessful Attempt

Learning phlebotomy skills is a psychomotor activity. This means that one's skill will improve over time and with practice. It also means that it is realistic to expect a lack of success now and again. Students must know how to react if a procedure is not successful in securing a specimen.

If the phlebotomist inserts the lancet into the patient's ear and the ear does NOT begin to bleed, the phlebotomist should:

1. Immediately discard the lancet into the appropriate needle disposal unit.
2. Discard all refuse and used materials (gauze, alcohol pads, etc) in the appropriate container.
3. Beginning at step 5 (select, prepare, and organize equipment) in Procedure 1, repeat the procedure. The procedure should be repeated using ALL new items. This means that a new lancet should be opened, as well as a new alcohol prep pad.
4. Students should limit their collection attempts to 2, unless otherwise directed by the instructor or supervisor.

Checklist: Duke Bleeding Time

(A) Performed **(B) Needs Improvement** **(C) Not Performed**

Comments:

______1. Washes hands.
______2. Dons gloves and gown.
______3. Role play: Approaches patient.
______4. Role play: Identifies patient, using the 2-step method of identification.
______5. Role play: Explains procedure to patient.
______6. Questions patient concerning medications he/she has taken during the past 7 to 10 days.
______7. Selects, prepares, and organizes equipment.
______8. Cleanses earlobe with alcohol.

Comments: **(A) Performed** **(B) Needs Improvement** **(C) Not Performed**

_____ 9. Allows site to air dry.
_____ 10. Appropriately grasps earlobe.
_____ 11. Punctures earlobe with sterile lancet and simultaneously starts stopwatch.
_____ 12. Appropriately wicks blood from puncture site.
_____ 13. Observes for cessation of bleeding. Stops stopwatch.
_____ 14. Rounds time to nearest 30 seconds.
_____ 15. Records time on result sheet.
_____ 16. Disposes lancet in a needle disposal unit.
_____ 17. Disposes blood-contaminated waste in a biohazard container.
_____ 18. Disposes noncontaminated refuse in appropriate waste receptacles.
_____ 19. Removes all equipment from patient's vicinity.
_____ 20. Removes gloves.
_____ 21. Washes hands.
_____ 22. Leaves patient courteously.

Result Sheet:

Duke Bleeding Time

Patient name: ______________________________

Duke bleeding time result: ______________________________

Do the patient's bleeding time results fall within the normal range? __________

Explain. ______________________________

Study Questions
Lab 8

1. List the 3 components of hemostasis. ______________________________

2. What role do platelets have in hemostasis? ______________________________

3. Describe the effect of platelets on bleeding time results. ______________________________

4. What physiologic change in vivo activates the intrinsic pathway? ______________________________

5. What physiologic change in vivo activates the extrinsic pathway? ______________________________

6. Describe fibrinolysis in vivo. ______________________________

____

____

7. Is the Duke bleeding time used frequently for routine bleeding time testing?

____

____

8. A patient's bleeding time is abnormally prolonged. What might this indicate?

____

____

LAB 9

Modified Ivy Bleeding Time Procedure

Objective

To instruct the procedure for the modified Ivy bleeding time

Equipment

Gloves; Gown; 70% isopropyl alcohol prep pad; Filter paper; Stopwatch; Bleeding time instrument; Butterfly bandage; Needle disposal unit; Biohazard bag

History of the Procedure

In 1941, Ivy et al introduced the first major innovations for standardizing the bleeding time test. Ivy chose the forearm as the bleeding time site, and he applied a blood pressure cuff inflated to 40 mm Hg on the upper arm to control capillary tone and to improve both the sensitivity and reproducibility of the test. The **sensitivity** of a test refers to its ability to detect borderline abnormalities. The more sensitive a test is, the more likely it is to detect small deviations from normal. The **reproducibility** of a test refers to the reproducibility of the test results. If a test has high reproducibility, 2 persons performing the same procedure under identical circumstances will arrive at identical results.

In 1969, Mielke and colleagues modified the Ivy bleeding time. They introduced a template. The template standardized the length and depth of a "surgical" incision made with a scalpel blade. The advantages of the template/scalpel included the following: the "surgical" incision more closely approximated the patient's hemostatic response to surgery, when compared to the puncture wound made in the Ivy procedure; the large surface area of the template minimized skin displacement; and the depth of the incision could be controlled.

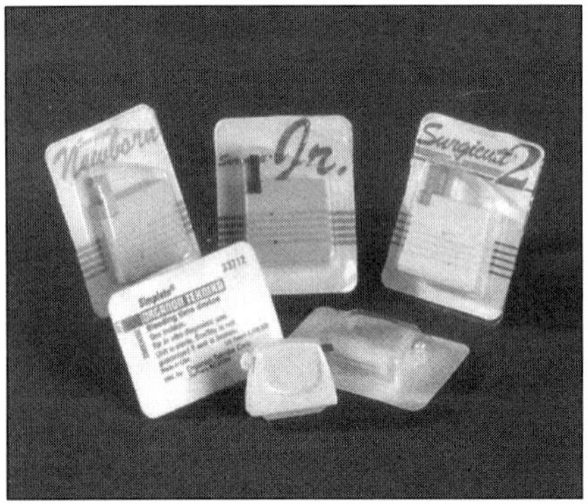

Figure 9-1 Automated incision-making devices.

The procedure introduced by Mielke et al was not widely used because the scalpel and template required sterilization after each use. In addition, the unconcealed scalpel caused patient apprehension, which was unpleasant for both the patient and the person performing the procedure. In 1978, a bleeding time device was made commercially available. The first bleeding time device introduced was the Simplate® (General Diagnostics, Division of Organon Teknika). The scalpel blade used by Mielke et al was replaced with a razor blade and the template was replaced with the flat narrow edge of the device. These devices make standardized incisions and are also sterile, disposable, and relatively inexpensive.

Bleeding Time Device

In addition to the Simplate®, several automated incision-making instruments for bleeding times are currently on the market (**Fig. 9-1**). The incision instruments are housed in plastic units, which are used once and then discarded. Normal values will depend on the bleeding time instrument chosen. Consult your instructor for the normal values associated with the bleeding time instrument selected for use at your facility.

Clinical Significance

The clinical significance of the modified Ivy bleeding time is the same as the Duke bleeding time (see Lab #8). Results of the modified Ivy bleeding time may also be affected if the patient has ingested aspirin or aspirin-containing compounds 7 to 10 days prior to the test.

Because the results of the modified Ivy bleeding time are more reliable and reproducible, the modified Ivy bleeding time has been substituted for the Duke bleeding time as the procedure of choice in many institutions.

Quality Assurance

1. Blood pressure cuffs must be appropriately applied to the patient's arm. The gauge should be maintained at 40 mm Hg throughout the procedure.
2. To ensure accurate, reproducible results, the length, depth, and direction of the bleeding time device must be standardized.

   Incision lengths of 5 to 9 mm afford similar results. If the length is shortened to 3 mm, the bleeding time is shortened. Although the bleeding time is shortened, the results are reproducible and sensitive. The choice of bleeding time instrument determines the length of the incision. The most common length used is 5 mm.

   Incision depth is critical to the accuracy of bleeding time results. The incision should be superficial so only capillaries and small blood vessels are involved. A depth of 1 mm is recommended. All commercially prepared bleeding time instruments are gauged to make incisions 1 mm deep. The phlebotomist should exercise care not to exert pressure on the bleeding time device while making the incision. With even slight pressure, significant indentation of the skin can occur. Such indentation may result in an incision greater than 1 mm deep.

Incisions made horizontally or vertically will yield reproducible results. It is imperative for reproducible results that everyone at a facility position the bleeding time device in the same direction. Incisions made horizontally to the antecubital crease are somewhat more sensitive to the effects of aspirin and/or borderline abnormalities in the primary hemostatic mechanism. An incision made horizontally is consistent with the direction of skin lines on the forearm; therefore, a cosmetic advantage is achieved with a horizontal position.

3. The action of cleansing the site before making the incision must be gentle. Vigorous cleaning may induce hyperemia, which is an excessive accumulation of blood at the puncture site.
4. Be sure not to touch the incision with the filter paper. If the incision is disturbed during the wicking process, adhering platelets may become dislodged, resulting in a falsely prolonged bleeding time. A diminishing blood flow followed by sudden resurgence in bleeding may indicate such an occurrence.

Procedure: Modified Ivy Bleeding Time

1. Wash hands. Don gloves and gown.

2. Role play: Approach patient. The interaction between patient and phlebotomist will be very similar to the interaction that takes place prior to the Duke bleeding time (refer to Lab #8).

3. Role play: Identify the patient, following the 2-step method of identification.

4. Role play: Explain the procedure to the patient. Interview the patient concerning aspirin-containing compounds.

5. Select, prepare, and organize equipment.

6. Position the sphygmomanometer cuff above the antecubital crease.

7. Secure the sphygmomanometer cuff.

8. Inspect the lateral aspect, volar surface of the forearm, approximately 5 cm below the antecubital crease for site selection. The following considerations should be made in site selection: the arm should not be edematous or paralyzed; the arm should be free of intravenous lines and shunts; the site should not be calloused or scarred; and the site should be free of blood vessels.
9. Cleanse the site selected by moving the alcohol pad in concentric circles from the incision site outward.
10. Turn the knob on the bulb of the sphygmomanometer until it stops. Squeeze the bulb to inflate the sphygmomanometer. Inflate the blood pressure cuff to 40 mm Hg.
11. Apply the bleeding time device to the incision site. The puncture must be performed within 30 to 60 seconds of inflation of the blood pressure cuff.
12. Depress the "trigger" on the bleeding time device without pressing down on the skin. Simultaneously start the stopwatch.
13. Using the filter paper, absorb the blood from the incision. Be careful NOT to touch the wound with the filter paper.
14. When the site has stopped bleeding (indicated by the absence of blood on the filter paper), stop the stopwatch.
15. Release the blood pressure cuff by turning the knob next to the bulb in the opposite direction used to inflate the cuff. Remove the blood pressure cuff.
16. Using sterile gauze and water, reclean the incision site. Dry the site, using sterile gauze.
17. Remove a butterfly bandage from its packaging.
18. Apply the tape from one end of the bandage to one side of the incision.
19. Pulling the tape so the edges of the incision meet together, apply the tape from the second side of the bandage.
20. Record the time on the stopwatch onto the requisition.
21. Dispose of waste materials in the appropriate receptacles (refer to Lab #8).

Checklist: **(A) Performed** **(B) Needs Improvement** **(C) Not Performed**

Modified Ivy Bleeding Time

Comments:

_____ 1. Washes hands before starting the procedure.
_____ 2. Dons gloves and gown.
_____ 3. Role play: Approaches patient.
_____ 4. Role play: Identifies the patient, using the 2-step method of patient identification.
_____ 5. Role play: Explains the procedure to the patient.
_____ 6. Role play: Questions patient concerning medications he/she has taken over the past 7 to 10 days.
_____ 7. Selects, prepares, and organizes equipment.
_____ 8. Selects site for bleeding time.
_____ 9. Positions the blood pressure cuff.
_____ 10. Cleanses the incision site.
_____ 11. Applies bleeding time device to the incision site.
_____ 12. Inflates the blood pressure cuff to 40 mm Hg.
_____ 13. Makes incision, simultaneously starts stopwatch.
_____ 14. Appropriately wicks flow of blood from incision.
_____ 15. Observes for the cessation of bleeding. Stops stopwatch when bleeding has ceased.
_____ 16. Releases gauge on blood pressure cuff.
_____ 17. Removes blood pressure cuff.
_____ 18. Recleanses the incision site.
_____ 19. Applies butterfly bandage.
_____ 20. Records time on requisition.
_____ 21. Disposes bleeding time instrument in needle disposal unit.
_____ 22. Disposes materials contaminated with blood in the biohazard bag.

_____ 23. Disposes noncontaminated waste in appropriate waste receptacles.
_____ 24. Removes all equipment from patient's vicinity.
_____ 25. Removes gloves.
_____ 26. Washes hands.
_____ 27. Leaves patient courteously.

Result Sheet:

Modified Ivy Bleeding Time

Patient name: ______________________________

Modified Ivy bleeding time result: ______________________________

Do the patient's bleeding time results fall within the normal range? ______________

Explain. ______________________________

____

____

Study Questions
Lab 9

1. A phlebotomist interviews a patient prior to performing a modified Ivy bleeding time test. The phlebotomist discovers that the patient took several doses of Coricidin over a 3-day period 5 days previously. What is the appropriate course of action for the phlebotomist? ______________________________

____

2. What is the most critical aspect of the bleeding time procedure for reproducible results? ______________________________

3. Draw the cascade concept of coagulation. Be sure to include the intrinsic, extrinsic, and common pathways.

4. Draw the fibrinolytic mechanism.

LAB 10

Venipuncture of the Artificial Arms

Objective

To introduce and familiarize the student with the venipuncture procedure

Equipment

Gloves; Gown; Artificial arm; 70% isopropyl alcohol prep pads; 2 x 2-inch gauze pads or cotton balls; Tourniquet; Holder; Needle; Evacuated tubes; Needle disposal unit; Biohazard bag

Discussion

Performing venipuncture is both a learned skill and an art. The learned skill of venipuncture refers to the steps incorporated into the procedure. To learn the skill, phlebotomists must learn which equipment to select, the steps in the procedure, and quality control procedures. The art of venipuncture rests in the phlebotomist's ability to interact professionally with the patient and to perform the procedures as painlessly as possible. Performing a "painless" venipuncture is truly an art form! Obviously, every patient wishes to have blood drawn by a person who is competent in phlebotomy techniques (the learned skill) and who also possesses kindness and compassion for patients and is striving to perfect the technique to achieve the painless venipuncture (the art). This lab is designed to assist the student in perfecting the learned skill, venipuncture. By the completion of this exercise, the student should be confident in EVERY STEP of the venipuncture procedure. In Lab #16, the art of venipuncture will be addressed.

In the previous labs, the following tasks common to most phlebotomy procedures were introduced: handwashing, quality control, patient identification, patient approach, and appropriate disposal of waste materials. This lab introduces another task common to EVERY specimen collection procedure: labeling.

Labeling

Following collection of a blood specimen, the specimen must be appropriately labeled. Proper patient identification and accurate labeling of patient specimens are the 2 most important quality control procedures for quality specimen collection. In Lab #6, proper patient identification was discussed. The corollary to proper patient identification is proper labeling of patient specimens. A blood specimen collected from the appropriate patient is not useful if it is labeled with another patient's name and information. If a specimen is mislabeled with incorrect patient information, the test results may be reported on the wrong patient, possibly compromising care. Inappropriate treatments may have disastrous consequences for the patient. Labeling information required on patient specimens will vary from facility to facility, and procedures are detailed in every facility's procedure manual.

There are 2 methods of generating a label. The first method is by computer. If labels are computer generated, the computer will print all of the required patient information on the label. The phlebotomist should always double-check the label information generated by the computer against that on the requisition to ensure that the information matches exactly. The only data the phlebotomist must write on a computer-generated label are the date and time of specimen collection and the phlebotomist's initials.

The second method of generating a label is by manually transposing (writing) required patient information onto a label. Information required on manually labeled specimens may include the following:

Patient's Name: The patient's first and last name should appear on specimen labels. Neither the first name nor the last name should be represented with an initial.

Patient's Identification Number: When a patient is admitted to the hospital, a hospital identification number is issued. Every patient has a different hospital identification number. If 2 patients in the hospital have the same name, their identities may be distinguished and confirmed using their hospital identification numbers. Patient identification numbers should appear on all specimen labels.

Inpatient Room and Bed Number: The patient's location within a health care facility may be indicated with a room and bed number (eg, 210W–2 [room 210 west, bed 2] or 330–5 [room 330, bed 5]).

Date and Time of Specimen Collection: The date and time of specimen collection may be required on the label. The date should include the month, day, and year (eg, 5/25/92). The time should reflect the time of day the sample was collected (eg, 8:20 PM or 2020).

Phlebotomist's Initials: The phlebotomist should initial every tube he/she collects. If there is a question concerning collection of the specimen, the person who collected it may be identified and consulted.

Labels should be affixed to blood specimen tubes immediately after collecting the specimen and before leaving the patient's side. Labels should be affixed vertically on the tube—not surrounding the tube—so the technologist can easily view the contents of the tube.

Inpatient vs Outpatient

The labeling guidelines above apply to inpatients. Inpatients are those patients who have been admitted to the hospital and assigned a bed. Inpatients will remain in the hospital for at least 1 night. Outpatients are patients who come to the hospital for a test or treatment and return home. Identification and labeling procedures for outpatients vary from inpatient identification and labeling procedures because most outpatients do not have a hospital identification bracelet affixed to their wrist.

To identify outpatients, some facilities incorporate the use of a medical records number. A patient's medical records number is assigned once and used whenever the patient has a transaction with that health care facility, either as an inpatient or an outpatient. Outpatient identification may be accomplished using the patient's medical records number as a secondary source of patient identification and should appear on outpatient specimen labels.

If a health care facility does not incorporate the use of a medical records number as a source of patient identification, outpatients may be identified by home address or social security number. Most facilities do not require a patient's address and/or social security number on the label of outpatient specimens. The outpatient specimen is simply marked "OP."

Procedural Issues

Successful venipuncture will depend to a large extent on how well the chosen vein is anchored. To adequately anchor a vein, place the thumb of your left hand (persons who are left-handed should use their right thumb) on the vein below the site selected for venipuncture. Place the index finger of the left hand (persons who are left-handed should use the index finger of their right hand) on the vein above the site selected for venipuncture. Gently push down on the vein selected, holding it in place until the needle has been inserted. Do NOT touch the back of the needle onto the glove of the thumb prior to insertion! This will contaminate the needle. If the thumb or index finger is removed before the needle is inserted, the vein will not be adequately anchored. This may lead to an unsuccessful venipuncture attempt.

When pushing tubes onto the needle, or removing tubes from the back of the needle, keep the holder ABSOLUTELY STILL. To accomplish this, rest the knuckles of the hand holding the evacuated tube apparatus on the patient's arm to help keep the holder securely in position. In addition, focus attention on either the point at which the needle is inserted into the arm or the plastic hub attachment to the holder. If the holder is NOT being held securely, the needle will move. If the needle is moving during the venipuncture procedure, the phlebotomist must make adjustments on the holder to maintain the position of the needle.

Quality Control

Specific quality control issues related to the venipuncture procedure will be addressed comprehensively in Lab #16. However, one quality control issue must be introduced at this time. Before using a needle, the phlebotomist must inspect the seal of the needle to ensure that it is intact before placing the needle onto the holder. If the seal is broken—or appears suspect in any way—the phlebotomist should discard the needle in a needle disposal unit and select another needle for use. If the seal of a needle is compromised, the phlebotomist must assume that the needle is unsterile and dispose of it appropriately.

Before inserting the needle into a patient's arm, the phlebotomist should visually inspect the needle for any sign of manufacturing defects, such as burrs or hooks (**Fig. 4-3**). Obviously, if the phlebotomist observes any manufacturing defects, the needle should be discarded in a needle disposal unit. Another needle should be selected for use.

Quality test results depend heavily on proper patient identification and preparation. The student phlebotomist should "interview" the artificial arm to determine both the patient's identity and the patient's adherence to preparation guidelines. Not all laboratory tests have special patient preparation guidelines. In fact, most do not. However, the phlebotomist must remember to screen the patient regarding these guidelines whenever appropriate.

Procedure 1: Venipuncture of Artificial Arms

1. Attend instructor's demonstration on the operation of the artificial arms.
2. Wash hands. Don gloves and gown.
3. Role play: Approach the patient. Identify yourself, the department you represent, and the procedure you are about to perform. ("Hello, my name is_____. I'm from the lab, and I'm here to collect a blood specimen for a test your physician has ordered.")
4. Role play: Identify the patient following the 2-step method of identification.
5. Role play: Explain the procedure to the patient. Most patients have previously had their blood drawn. An appropriate question to address this issue might be, "Have you ever had your blood drawn before?" If the patient has never had blood collected before, the phlebotomist should explain the procedure before proceeding. Interview the patient concerning patient preparation guidelines, if appropriate. (Your lab partner should respond for the artificial arm!)
6. Select the equipment. Prepare the evacuated tube system. Inspect the seal of the needle. Be sure the seal is intact before using the needle. Affix the needle to the holder. Position the evacuated tube selected into the back of the holder. Some phlebotomists like to partially pierce the stopper with the needle (see **Fig. 10-2,** right). This facilitates pushing the tube onto the back of the needle once the needle is in the vein. Push the evacuated tube onto the stopper until the stopper reaches the line on the holder. Organize the equipment in order of use during the procedure.
7. Secure tourniquet (refer to Lab #7).
8. Select a venipuncture site by palpating for a vein (refer to Lab #7).

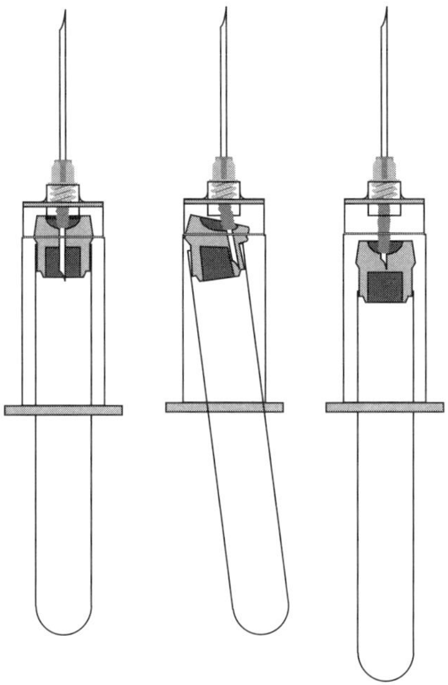

Figure 10-2 Left, proper insertion of evacuated tube into holder; middle, improper insertion resulting in a completely punctured stopper; right, partially punctured stopper.

9. Release the tourniquet.
10. Cleanse the site with 70% alcohol prep pad. Begin at the puncture site selected and move the alcohol pad outward, in concentric circles.
11. Allow the area to air dry.
12. Reapply the tourniquet. Be sure the ends do not touch the prepared site.
13. Position the holder between your thumb and index finger. Your palm should be pointing to the left if you are right-handed, and to the right if you are left-handed.
14. Uncap the needle. Inspect the needle for manufacturer's defects.
15. Anchor the vein selected, using the thumb and index finger.
16. Position the needle in the same direction as the vein selected. Insert the needle, bevel up, at a 15-degree angle. The needle should be inserted in 1 smooth motion. Only the index finger and thumb should move forward to glide the needle into the vein.
17. Release the vein, and push the evacuated tube onto the back of the needle (**Fig. 10-2**). Be sure to keep the holder stationary. Once the tube has been pushed onto the needle, take your hand off of the tube. If the stopper of the tube has been punctured by the back of the needle, and blood is not entering the tube, pushing on the tube will NOT cause blood to enter it.
18. Allow the tube to fill. When the vacuum has been exhausted, blood will no longer enter the tube.
19. Keeping the holder absolutely still, pull the evacuated tube off the back of the needle and replace it with the second tube. (If the first tube contained an additive, you may gently invert it while waiting for the second tube to fill.)
20. Once blood begins to enter the second tube, release the tourniquet within 1 minute of application.
21. Pull the evacuated tube off of the needle. Allow it to rest in the holder.
22. Place a piece of gauze (or cotton) over the puncture site. Do not push down on the gauze.
23. Remove the needle.

24. Remove the evacuated tube from the holder and discard the needle into a needle disposal unit.
25. If the evacuated tube contains an additive, invert gently several times to mix the blood with the additive.
26. Inspect puncture site. Apply bandage, if needed.
27. Label the tubes collected IMMEDIATELY following collection (refer to the discussion section of this lab).
28. Record specimen on result sheet.
29. Discard materials contaminated with blood in the biohazard bag.
30. Remove gloves.
31. Wash hands.
32. Leave patient courteously.

Procedure 2: Unsuccessful Attempt

Venipuncture of the artificial arms is a learned skill. Therefore, it is unrealistic to expect to complete the 30 assigned draws in 30 attempts. Students must know how to react if a procedure is not successful in securing a specimen.

If the phlebotomist does not achieve blood flow into the evacuated tube, the phlebotomist should:

1. Untie the tourniquet.
2. Remove the evacuated tube from the back of the needle.
3. Place gauze over the puncture site.
4. Withdraw the needle.
5. Immediately place the needle into a needle disposal unit.
6. Beginning at step #6 above, repeat the procedure.

Some of the most common errors that lead to unsuccessful venipuncture attempts on the artificial arms are the following:

- **Failure to insert the needle completely into the vein.** The phlebotomist should feel resistance initially following insertion of the needle. The resistance is almost immediately followed by a sensation of free or easier movement of the needle. When the phlebotomist no longer senses the resistance, the needle is in the vein. Once the phlebotomist senses that the needle has been inserted into the vein, the evacuated tube should be pushed onto the needle—NOT before.

- **Puncturing the stopper before entering the vein.** If the phlebotomist partially pushes the evacuated tube onto the needle before inserting the needle into the vein, he/she risks puncturing the stopper and releasing the vacuum.
- **Malfunctioning of the artificial arm.** Sometimes the artificial arms do not function as expected. If the student suspects this to be the case, he/she should notify the instructor.

Result Sheet: Instructions

1. You must complete 30 venipunctures. A venipuncture will be considered complete only if it is initialed by the instructor and is accompanied by a completed checklist.
2. Of the 30 venipunctures assigned, 20 are to be completed as single draws and 10 as multidraws. A single draw is the collection of 1 evacuated tube. A multidraw is the collection of 2 evacuated tubes.
3. Stopper colors have been selected for you and are listed on your result sheet. Assign a test to each tube and complete the chart (see Appendix 2).
4. The sequence of collection of evacuated tubes in a multidraw should be in this order: 1) blood culture, 2) red top or SST, 3) blue top, 4) green top, 5) lavender, 6) black, and 7) gray.
5. Each venipuncture must be witnessed and evaluated by your lab partner or instructor, using the checklists.
6. Remember, the purpose of this exercise is to allow you to learn and develop good venipuncture technique. Don't be shy about calling your lab partner's attention to mistakes he/she made. Common mistakes students commit when learning venipuncture include the following: 1) *Retouching the site just before inserting the needle:* If you are going to repalpate, you must either cleanse your index finger before repalpating, or recleanse the site before

puncture. 2) *Not anchoring the vein before inserting the needle:* The vein must be held in place for successful needle penetration. 3) *"Bouncing" the needle on the skin before gliding it into the vein:* During venipuncture, the patient should only be stuck once with the needle. 4) *Not keeping the holder stationary:* For successful venipuncture, the holder must be held absolutely stationary so the needle is not dislodged from the vein.

The evaluator should be very critical of the phlebotomist's technique. Remember, the person practicing on the artificial arm today may be your phlebotomist in the future. React as though the artificial arm were your own!

Checklist:

Venipuncture of Artificial Arms

(A) Performed **(B) Needs Improvement** **(C) Not Performed**

Comments:

_____ 1. Washes hands before approaching patient.
_____ 2. Dons gloves and gown.
_____ 3. Role play: Approaches patient.
_____ 4. Role play: Performs 2-step identification of patient.
_____ 5. Role play: Explains procedure.
_____ 6. Selects equipment.
_____ 7. Prepares equipment (includes inspecting the seal of the needle).
_____ 8. Organizes equipment.
_____ 9. Positions patient's arm.
_____ 10. Applies tourniquet.
_____ 11. Uses index finger to palpate for a venipuncture site.
_____ 12. Releases tourniquet.
_____ 13. Cleanses venipuncture site by moving alcohol in concentric circles from puncture site outward.

Comments: **(A) Performed** **(B) Needs Improvement** **(C) Not Performed**

______14. Allows site to air dry.
______15. Reapplies tourniquet without contaminating venipuncture site.
______16. Positions evacuated tube holder; uncaps needle.
______17. Inspects needle for manufacturer's defects.
______18. Anchors vein with thumb and index finger.
______19. Inserts needle, bevel up, at correct angle.
______20. Inserts needle in same direction as the vein.
______21. Pushes evacuated tube onto needle, without moving the holder.
______22. Draws evacuated tubes in the appropriate order.
______23. Releases tourniquet.
______24. Removes last evacuated tube from the back of the needle.
______25. Places gauze over puncture site.
______26. Withdraws needle and discards immediately in a needle disposal unit.
______27. Gently inverts tubes with additives 5 to 10 times following the draw.
______28. Inspects puncture site. Applies bandage, if needed.
______29. Labels tube(s) with appropriate information.
______30. Labels tubes immediately following the draw.
______31. Discards materials contaminated with blood in the biohazard bag. Removes equipment.
______32. Removes gloves and washes hands.
______33. Leaves patient courteously.

Record Sheet 1:
Single Draws

Single Draw No.	Instructor's Initials	Patient's Name	Tests Ordered	Stopper Color(s)	Tube Additive	Department	Clinical Significance
1			Alkaline phosphatase				
2			ASAT				
3			CK				
4			Hemoglobin				
5			Reticulocyte				
6			Platelet count				
7			CRP				
8			ASO titer				
9			Heterophile				
10			Rubella				
11*			Glucose				
12*			D-Xylose				
13			Electrolytes				
14			LDH				
15			LDH isoenzyme				
16			Ammonia				
17			Osmotic fragility				
18			Sickle cell				
19			Total eosinophil				
20			G-6PD				

Multidraw No.	Instructor's Initials	Patient's Name	Tests Ordered	Stopper Color(s)	Tube Additive	Department	Clinical Significance
1			Antibody screen				
			Hemoglobin electrophoresis				
2			VDRL				
			Prothrombin time				
3*			Glucose				
			LE Prep				
4			BUN				
			APTT				
5			HCG				
			Febrile agglutinins				
6*			Complement				
			Glucose				
7*			RA screen				
			ESR				
8			Sodium				
			CBC				
9			Uric acid				
			Fibrinogen				
10			CBC				
			LE Prep				

* Tests requiring special patient preparation.

Study Questions
Lab 10

1. What is the rationale for the "order of draw" when multiple specimen tubes are collected from 1 patient?

2. List at least 6 departments found in most hospital or clinical laboratories. For each department, list 2 analyses commonly performed. Identify the collection tube most commonly delivered to each department.

3. Compare and contrast the following positions in the hospital or clinical laboratory: pathologist, medical technologist, medical laboratory technician, phlebotomist.

4. What qualifications are required for a person to be a department supervisor in the laboratory?

5. How are the CLIA '88 regulations expected to impact each position listed in questions 3 and 4 above?

LAB 11

Skin Punctures: Microhematocrit Determinations and ABO Blood Typing

Objective

To gain expertise in skin puncture technique

Equipment

70% isopropyl alcohol prep pads; Sterile gauze; Heel warmer; Blood lancet; Masks; Protective eyewear; Gown; Gloves; 3 capillary microhematocrit tubes: 2 plain (blue ring) and 1 heparinized (red ring); Typing sera: Anti-A and Anti-B; Blood typing slides; 2 applicator sticks; Sealing clay; Microhematocrit centrifuge; Microhematocrit tube reader; Needle disposal unit; Biohazard bag

Discussion

Skin puncture procedures are performed instead of venipuncture procedures primarily for 2 reasons: 1) the patient is an infant or small child, or 2) the specimen was unattainable by venipuncture.

This laboratory exercise is designed to introduce the student to the procedure for collecting a blood specimen by skin puncture for analyses that require a small amount of specimen.

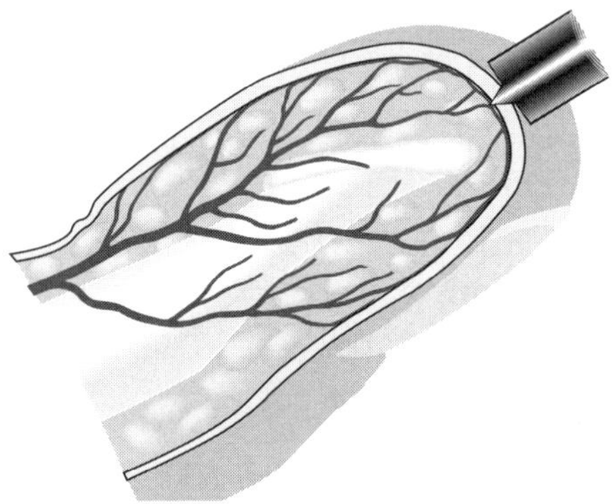

Figure 11-1 Proper depth of lancet for puncture.

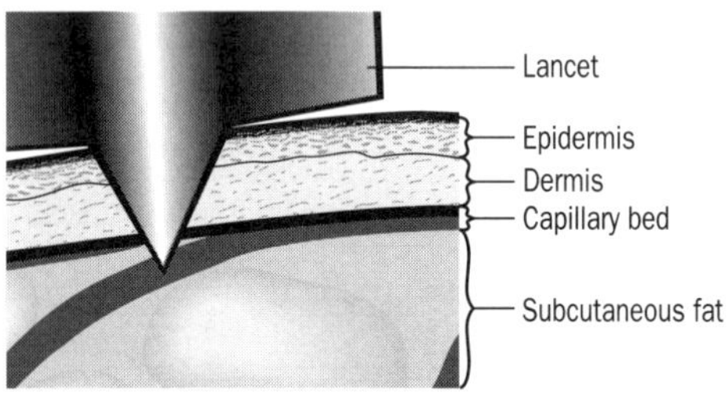

Figure 11-2 Lancet must puncture dermis and subcutaneous tissue to reach the capillary bed.

Adequate Puncture

When collecting blood specimens by skin puncture, performing a good puncture is critical to the success of the procedure. A good puncture will appropriately access capillaries, veins and arteries at the junction of the dermis and subcutaneous tissue (**Fig. 11-1, Fig. 11-2**). If the puncture is not performed properly, an inadequate number of capillaries, veins, and arteries will be accessed, and an insufficient volume of specimen will result. The first step in performing a good puncture is immobilizing the skin puncture site. Many times, patients will move their finger away from the lancet in a reflex motion. Unless the phlebotomist has secured the site, withdrawal of the site from the lancet will result in too shallow a puncture. In this lab, the patient's finger is the designated site. To adequately immobilize the site, place a digit (finger or thumb) on the patient's fingernail and a second digit on the pad of the patient's fingertip, just below the selected puncture site (see **Fig. 6-2**). Anchor your hand and the patient's finger on a hard surface, such as the arm of the phlebotomy chair.

The second step in performing a good puncture is proper lancet application. Hold the lancet between the thumb and index finger. While holding the patient's finger securely, position the lancet above the selected puncture site. The lancet should be positioned perpendicular to the patient's fingerprints and at almost a 90-degree angle to the puncture site (see **Fig. 6-5**). By moving the wrist in a direct, forward motion, the lancet should pierce the puncture site. Insert the entire point of the lancet during the puncture. If the lancet is not entirely inserted during puncture, an insufficient sample will result.

Insufficient Specimen (QNS)

If an insufficient quantity of specimen is obtained following a skin puncture, the puncture must be repeated. To repeat a skin puncture on the same patient, all materials used for the initial puncture must be discarded and new materials opened for use. This is especially true of the lancet. Lancets should be used for ONE puncture only! If an initial puncture is unsuccessful, the lancet is discarded in a needle disposal unit, and a new one is opened. In most instances, if a student is unsuccessful in securing a blood sample following skin puncture, it is the result of a shallow puncture. The corrective action is to repeat the puncture. To ensure a puncture of appropriate depth, the lancet must be inserted up to the guards (**Fig. 11-2**), and the site must be immobilized to allow the lancet to sufficiently penetrate the skin.

Collection of Specimen/ Capillary Tubes

The first drop of blood generated from a skin puncture site is NOT collected for analysis, since it may be contaminated with alcohol and tissue fluids, which may alter the values of lab results. Therefore, this first drop is wiped away with sterile gauze.

Hemolysis of a skin puncture specimen may be the result of residual alcohol on the skin. Alcohol causes red blood cells to rupture. Squeezing the heel or finger too hard can result in the mechanical rupturing of patient red blood cells. This is especially true of blood from newborns. Newborns have high hematocrit levels and fragile red blood cells, which make their blood specimens more susceptible to hemolysis.

To collect a skin puncture sample with a capillary tube (after the first drop of blood has been wiped away), position the tube between the thumb and index finger, with the palm of the hand underneath the capillary tube. The ring (blue or red) should be positioned away from the patient. Position a digit over the patient's fingernail and another on the pad of the patient's finger. Phlebotomists are often most successful if they apply pressure to the heel or finger with the dominant hand and position the collection tube in the other hand. Squeeze the finger. As blood begins to appear from the puncture site, apply the capillary tube to the blood. Do NOT touch the wound with the capillary tube! The blood will enter the tube by capillary action. Once the tube is three quarters filled or more, place your index finger over the tip of the tube with the ring, and place the blue-ringed tube into the sealing clay. Collect the next 2 tubes in the same manner, but do NOT seal the red-ringed tubes.

ABO Blood Typing

ABO blood typing is a procedure performed in the clinical laboratory to determine a patient's ABO blood type. The patient's ABO blood type will categorize the patient into 1 of 4 ABO blood groups: A, B, AB, or O. Of these 4 blood groups, A and O are the most common. Following is the percentage of persons in each group.

Incidence (%) of the ABO Blood Groups in Various Populations*

Race	A	B	AB	O
White	34–38	12–13	5–6	42–46
Black	19–27	21–23	3–6	45–48
Chinese	27–33	25–28	5–9	31–43

The range of reported values is derived from various studies.

*Reprinted with permission. Stansfield WD. *Serology & Immunology: A Clinical Approach.* New York, NY: Macmillan Publishing Co; 1981.

People in different blood groups have different factors on their red blood cell membranes. The factors are referred to by a variety of terms, including antigen, specificity, and determinant. Group A persons have A antigens on their red blood cells; group B persons have B antigens on their red blood cells; group AB persons have A and B antigens on their red blood cells; and group O persons have neither A nor B antigens on their red blood cells.

The antigens on a person's red blood cells can be identified by reacting the patient's red blood cells with an antiserum with known specificity (ie, the antiserum will react with a particular antigen and no other). For this lab, the antiserums selected for use are A (blue) and B (yellow). The A antiserum will react with A antigens on the red blood cells, and the B antiserum will react with the B antigens. The reaction is evidenced by agglutination, or clumping of the red blood cells.

Characteristically, agglutination in an antiserum will look like chips of red suspended in a clear supernate of antiserum. If no reaction occurs (ie, the patient's red blood cells do not possess antigens that will react with the antiserum), the red blood cells will appear throughout the antiserum, and the antiserum will appear cloudy or turbid. In a negative reaction, the supernate of the antiserum will not appear clear.

Blood group antisera are usually manufactured from pooled sera, which means that the plasma from many different people is used to prepare the antisera. Consequently, the antisera must be treated as a body fluid capable of transmitting HBV and/or HIV. OSHA's instructions from the Office of Health Compliance Assistance requires persons to wear protective gowns, gloves, eye wear, and masks if splashes to skin or clothing are likely to occur. It is recommended that persons performing ABO typing by this procedure also wear this protective clothing.

Microhematocrits

Microhematocrit determinations are usually performed in physician's offices or in blood bank donor rooms and are used to screen for anemia. The patient's whole blood is collected in a capillary tube and centrifuged. The packed cell volume following centrifugation is measured and expressed as a percentage. Normal ranges for microhematocrits in adults are 36% to 46% for women and 42% to 52% for men. Values lower than the normal range may indicate anemia in a patient. Abnormally elevated hematocrit levels may be caused by environmental factors, such as living in regions of high altitudes. High hematocrit levels may also be associated with a condition known as polycythemia, which is an abnormal increase in the number of erythrocytes.

Procedure 1: Skin Puncture

1. Wash hands. Don gloves and gown.
2. Role play: Approach patient. Explain the procedure (if necessary).
3. Role play: Identify the patient.
4. Select, prepare, and organize equipment (refer to Lab #8).
5. Select area for puncture site.
6. Gently massage finger chosen from hand to fingertip 3 to 4 times.
7. If the patient's hand is cold, apply a heel warmer to the skin puncture site.
8. Remove alcohol prep pad from package.
9. Cleanse the site, using a circular motion, beginning at the puncture site and moving outward.
10. Allow the site to air dry.
11. Hold the patient's finger securely.
12. Position the lancet above the puncture site, perpendicular to the fingerprints.
13. Puncture the site selected with one fluid motion. Try to insert the entire lancet point during the puncture.
14. Squeeze the finger to create a drop of blood at the puncture site.
15. Wipe the first drop of blood from the puncture site, using sterile gauze.
16. Collect blood in the 3 capillary tubes.
17. Once sample collection is completed, use a gauze pad to apply pressure to the puncture site until the bleeding stops. (Patients may be willing to do this themselves.) If the adult patient desires a bandage, affix the bandage over the puncture site. Do NOT affix bandages to skin puncture sites of young children. They may remove the bandage, place it in their mouths, and aspirate it.
18. Discard lancet in needle disposal unit.
19. Discard materials contaminated with blood in the biohazard bag.
20. Dispose of other waste materials in the appropriate receptacles.

Procedure 2: Blood Typing

1. Don protective eye wear, mask, gown, and gloves.
2. Place 2 drops of anti-A (blue serum) in one trough on the blood typing tray.
3. Place 2 drops of anti-B (yellow serum) in a second trough on the blood typing tray.
4. Place your finger over the end of the red-ringed capillary tube.
5. Position the tube over the first trough. Remove your finger from the end of the tube and allow one drop of blood to fall into the typing serum. Repeat with the second typing serum.
6. Using an applicator stick, mix the blood samples with the typing sera.
7. Tilt the blood typing tray back and forth for 2 minutes.
8. Observe for the presence (+) or absence (–) of agglutination (clumping of red blood cells).
9. Record the results on the result sheet.
10. Interpret the results, using the chart below:
11.

Anti-A	Anti-B	Blood Group
+	–	A
+	+	AB
–	+	B
–	–	O

Record the interpretation on the result sheet.

12. Discard waste materials and clean work area per your instructor's directions.

Procedure 3: Microhematocrit

1. Don protective eye wear, masks, gown, and gloves.
2. Seal the end of the blue-ringed capillary tubes with sealing clay.
3. Place the sealed capillary tubes in the microhematocrit centrifuge.
4. Position the capillary tubes exactly opposite each other, with the sealed end pointing to the outside rim of the centrifuge.
5. Centrifuge for the length of time designated by your instructor. (Timing will vary with the model of centrifuge.)
6. Read the results, using the microhematocrit tube reader.
7. Record the results on the result sheet.

Checklist: Skin Puncture

(A) Performed **(B) Needs Improvement** **(C) Not Performed**

Comments:

______1. Washes hands.
______2. Dons gloves, masks, eyewear, and gown.
______3. Role play: Approaches patient.
______4. Role play: Identifies patient, using the 2-step method of identification.
______5. Selects equipment.
______6. Prepares equipment.
______7. Organizes equipment.
______8. Selects site for skin puncture.
______9. Applies warmer to site when appropriate.
______10. Cleanses skin puncture site with alcohol.
______11. Allows site to air dry.
______12. Secures puncture site appropriately.
______13. Punctures site with lancet at the appropriate angle.
______14. Wipes away the first drop of blood.
______15. Applies pressure to the puncture site to collect an adequate sample.
______16. Collects tests in the appropriate order.
______17. Upon completion of collection, applies pressure to the puncture site, using sterile gauze, until the bleeding has stopped.

______18. Disposes lancet in the needle disposal unit.
______19. Discards materials contaminated with blood in the biohazard bag.
______20. Removes all equipment from the patient's vicinity.
______21. Inspects puncture site; applies bandage, if needed.
______22. Removes gloves.
______23. Washes hands.
______24. Leaves patient courteously.

Result Sheet: Blood Typing

Patient:
Results:
Anti-A:__________________ Anti-B:__________________

Interpretation (ABO blood group of patient):

____

Result Sheet: Microhematocrit

Patient:____________________________________

Slot numbers	Results (%)
__________	__________
__________	__________

The results should be $\pm$2% of each other. If your results vary by more than 2%, give a possible explanation. ______________________________

____

Inspect the serum in the microhematocrit tubes for hemolysis. Is hemolysis present?

____

If hemolysis is present, what is a possible explanation for its presence?________

____

Study Questions

Lab 11

1. What is a CBC? Which laboratory departments perform CBC analyses? ______

2. What tests are routinely included in a CBC analysis? ______

3. List at least 3 different instruments capable of analyzing a blood specimen for CBC. ______

4. What is immunohematology? What is the difference between immunohematology and transfusion services? ______

5. What percentage of the population has an Rh-negative blood type? What is the difference between Rh-negative and Rh-positive blood? ______

6. Would it be possible to determine a person's Rh type using the blood typing method employed in this lab? Why or why not? ______

LAB 12

Preparation of a Blood Smear

Objective

To introduce the glass slide (slide wedge) method of preparing a blood film

Equipment

Gloves; Gown; 3 glass slides, 25 x 75 mm (1 x 3 inches); Applicator sticks; EDTA blood sample; Paper toweling; Needle disposal unit; Biohazard bag

Discussion

A significant percentage of the work performed in the hematology laboratory involves assessing the morphology of blood cells. A drop of blood is smeared on a glass slide, stained, and examined underneath a microscope. Blood smears may be used in the following procedures:

1. Complete blood cell counts: differential white blood cell count; assessment of red blood cell morphology; platelet count estimation; and assessment of platelet morphology
2. Reticulocyte count
3. Confirmatory studies/manual platelet counts

The quality of test results in analyses incorporating the use of a blood smear will be greatly affected by the quality of the smear used for analysis.

Historically, the blood smear was prepared manually at the patient's bedside or at the outpatient draw station at the time of specimen collection. Each smear was transported to the hematology laboratory, stained, and examined under the microscope by the technologist. Recently, advances in technology offer instruments that prepare, stain, and read blood smears automatically. These advances have markedly reduced the number of blood smears prepared by the phlebotomy team.

Certain situations (eg, facilities without automated instrumentation, such as a physician's office laboratory or a small clinic) and procedures (eg, collection of a complete blood cell count following skin puncture using the Unopette® system) still require the preparation of blood smears at the patient's bedside.

Procedural Issues

The slide wedge procedure uses three 25 x 75-mm slides: 2 sample slides and 1 spreader slide. A blood smear is prepared on each of the glass slides, using the spreader slide. Characteristics of a good blood smear prepared by the slide wedge procedure include the following: 1) the smear should have a smooth, even surface with no ridges, waves, or holes; 2) the smear should not extend to the end of the slide, but should cover approximately one half to two thirds of the sample slide; 3) the smear should not cover the entire width of the slide, but a gap should exist on each side of the smear; 4) the smear should have a thick portion near the drop of blood and decrease in thickness, until it becomes a feathery edge toward the opposite end of the slide; and 5) the smear should end in a “feathered edge,” not in a straight line and with no “tails” extending off the end of the slide (**Fig. 12-1**).

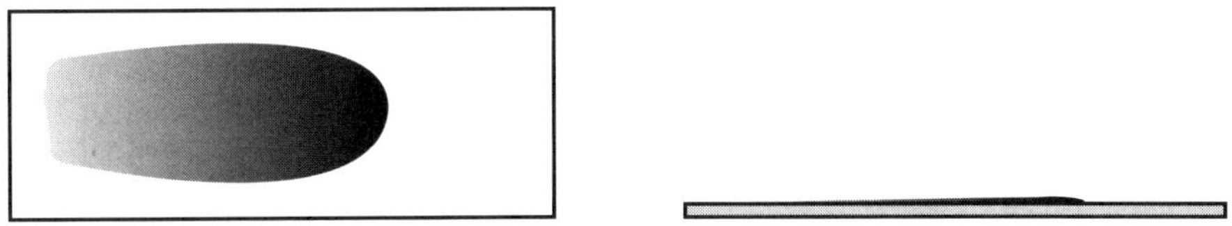

Figure 12-1 Top and side views of a properly prepared blood smear.

Common Problems

The ability to consistently prepare quality blood smears is acquired by practicing the technique. Common problems associated with the preparation of a quality blood film and the causes of those problems are listed in the following chart.

Problem	Possible Source of Error
Holes in the smear	• Dirty slide
Smear too thin	• Drop of blood too small • Angle of spreader slide too small • Very low patient hematocrit
Smear too thick	• Drop of blood too large • Angle of spreader slide too big • Very high patient hematocrit
Smear ends in a straight line, instead of a feathered edge	• Spreader slide was stopped near the end of the sample slide, instead of pushed past the end of the sample slide
Smear ends with a number of "tails," instead of a feathered edge	• Spreader slide was pulled through the drop of blood, instead of just up to it • Dirty edge on the spreader slide • Spreader slide was turned, so the edge of it was lifted off the sample slide • Edge of the spreader slide was chipped
Smear contains ridges or waves	• Spreader slide was moved in an uneven or "jerky" motion • Too much pressure was exerted on the spreader slide as it was moved across the sample slide

Procedure:

Preparation of a Blood Smear

1. Put on gloves, gown, and any other protective clothing required at your facility for this procedure. Place the EDTA blood sample on a mixing rack.
2. Designate 2 slides to be used for blood smear preparation and 1 slide to be used as a spreader slide. Be sure that all 3 slides are *scrupulously* clean.
3. Remove the EDTA tube from the mixing rack.
4. Unstopper the EDTA tube following the safety guidelines at your facility.
5. Place the tube into a test tube rack.
6. Hold 2 applicator sticks together and dip them into the tube of blood.
7. By touching the 2 applicator sticks onto the glass slide, place a small drop of blood (approximately 1–2 mm in diameter) on the slide, next to—but not touching—the frosted edge (**Fig. 12-2**). If the slide does not have a frosted edge, place the drop of blood approximately 1 cm from the edge of the slide. The smear must be made immediately after placing the drop of blood on the slide. Any delay in preparing the smear may result in abnormal distribution of white blood cells, with many of the larger ones accumulating at the thin edge of the smear. In addition, the red blood cells may take on an abnormal "stacked coin" appearance, called rouleaux. Platelet clumping may also occur.
8. Place the slide on a flat surface with the drop of blood to the right. (Persons who are left-handed should position the drop of blood to the left.)

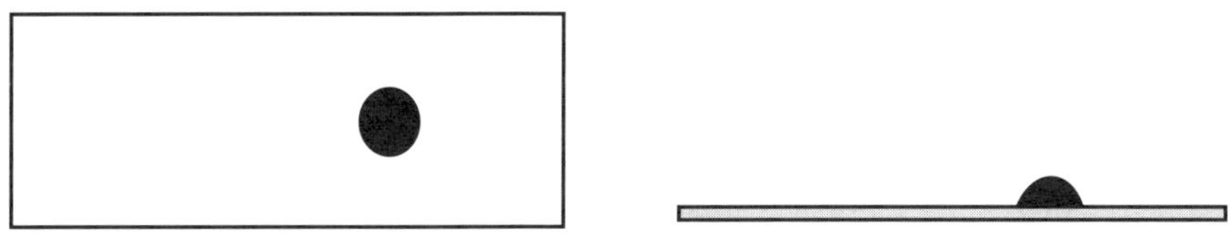

Figure 12-2 Top and side view of the relative size and placement of a drop of blood for a thin smear.

9. Position the spreader slide to the left of the drop of blood. (Persons who are left-handed should position the spreader slide to the right of the drop of blood.)
10. Tilt the spreader slide so the angle between the 2 slides approximates 25 to 30 degrees. Be sure only the edge of the spreader slide rests on the sample slide. Move the edge of the spreader slide toward the drop of blood. When the edge of the spreader slide contacts the drop of blood, stop moving the spreader slide.
11. Allow the blood to spread along the edge of the spreader slide.
12. Maintaining the spreader slide at a 25- to 30-degree angle, push the spreader slide away from the drop of blood (**Fig. 12-3**). Push the spreader slide all the way off the sample slide. Do NOT stop moving the spreader slide until it has gone beyond the end of the sample slide.
13. Repeat the procedure on the second sample slide. Use a clean edge of the spreader slide to make the second smear.
14. Allow the smears to air dry.
15. Label the smears. If the slide has a frosted edge, use a pencil to write the labeling information on the frosted edge. If the slide has no frosted edge, write the labeling information on a paper label and affix the label to the thick edge of the smear.

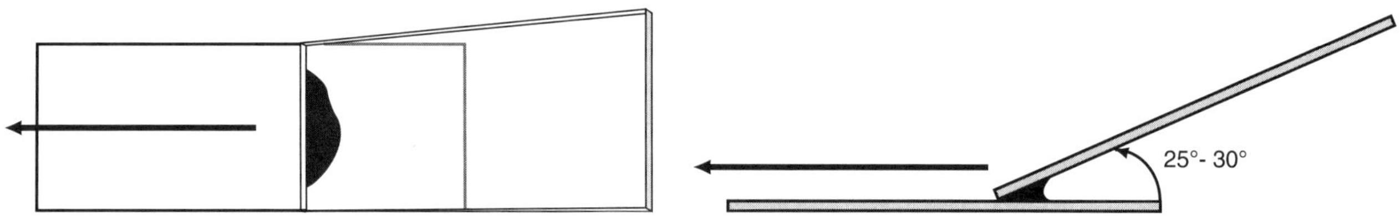

Figure 12-3 Top and side view of the position of the spreader slide in relation to the drop of blood.

16. Present the labeled smears to your instructor. The smears will be evaluated, using the checklist.
17. Remove protective clothing. Dispose in the appropriate waste receptacle.
18. Wash hands.

Checklist:

Preparation of a Blood Smear

Comments:

Prepare 2 blood smears, using the slide wedge technique. Your instructor must be satisfied with the quality of the smears. Most students must make several attempts at the procedure before generating 2 acceptable smears. Any unacceptable smears or contaminated spreader slides and applicator sticks must be discarded in a needle disposal unit. The area used to prepare the smears must be cleansed at the end of the lab session with an appropriate disinfectant.

A properly prepared blood smear has the following characteristics:

	Smear 1	Smear 2	
1.	________	________	Has a smooth, even surface.
2.	________	________	Has a thick portion, which tapers off into a thin portion.
3.	________	________	Ends in a feathered edge.
4.	________	________	Covers one half to two thirds of the slide.
5.	________	________	Has an appropriate thickness (is neither too thick nor too thin).
6.	________	________	Has a space on either side of the smear.
7.	________	________	Is appropriately labeled.

Study Questions
Lab 12

1. Compare and contrast the coverslip method of blood smear preparation and the slide wedge method of blood smear preparation. What are the advantages and disadvantages of each method?

2. A phlebotomist has requisitions for the following tests: platelet count, CBC, and electrolytes. The tests were ordered on a newborn baby. The microcollection method used requires the preparation of blood smears at the patient's bedside. In what order should the tests, including the blood smear, be collected?

3. What is the rationale for the order of draw used in question #2 above?

4. List 3 instruments capable of preparing blood smears.

5. List 3 instruments capable of performing automated WBC differential counts.

LAB 13
Introduction to Unopettes®

Objective

To introduce the concept of dilution as it applies to the Unopette® system; to properly use the Unopette® system to prepare dilutions of patient specimens; to gain expertise in performing skin puncture procedures

Equipment

70% isopropyl alcohol prep pads; Sterile gauze;
Heel warmer; Blood lancet; Gloves; Gown; 4 Unopette® systems;
4 blank labels; EDTA blood sample;
Tissue paper; Needle disposal unit;
Biohazard bag

Discussion

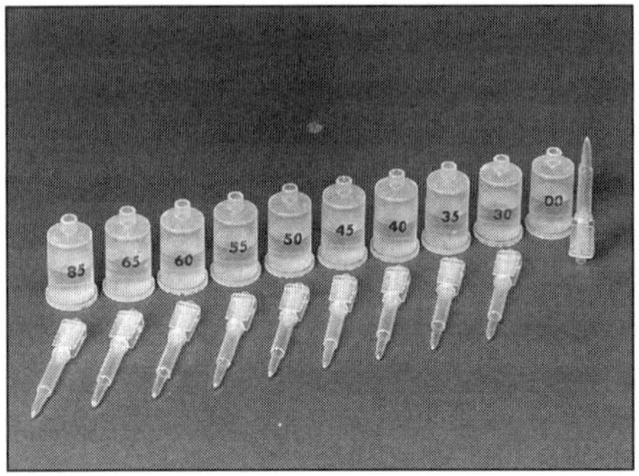

Figure 13-1 The Unopette® system. (Photo courtesy of Becton Dickinson)

When a patient's blood sample is diluted, the concentration of its elements is reduced. By reducing the concentration of a blood sample, counting the cellular elements of that sample is simplified. It is easier to count cellular elements of the blood once they have been diluted, because following dilution there are fewer elements to count. After counting the cellular elements of a diluted sample, the result is multiplied by a number, called the "dilution factor," to determine the result. The dilution factor is based on the ratio of amount of specimen to the amount of diluent. For example, if equal parts of specimen and diluent are mixed, the dilution factor is 2.

The Unopette® system provides a method of fast, easy, and accurate dilution of a patient's blood sample (**Fig. 13-1**). The Unopette® system is composed of a reservoir (containing the diluent), a pipette (calibrated to deliver a specific amount of blood to the reservoir), and a bullet shield (protects the pipette and is used to prepare the reservoir prior to dilution). Accurate dilutions require that specific amounts of a sample be added to specific amounts of a diluent. Accurate Unopette® dilutions require that specific amounts of patient blood sample be added to the diluent in the reservoir. Accurate Unopette® dilutions also require that the amount of diluent in the reservoir does not change.

Procedural Issues

The pipettes used with the Unopette® System are calibrated to deliver an exact amount of blood to the reservoir containing the diluent. To ensure that the pipette will deliver an exact amount of blood to the reservoir, the following conditions must be met:

1. The pipette must be filled to its neck (**Fig. 13-2a**). Underfilling or overfilling the pipette will affect the dilution (**Fig. 13-2b**).
2. The pipette cannot contain air bubbles (**Fig. 13-2c**). Air bubbles in the blood sample collected in the pipette will reduce the amount of blood delivered to the diluent, altering the blood:diluent ratio. If the blood:diluent ratio is altered, the test results become significantly altered and no longer accurate.

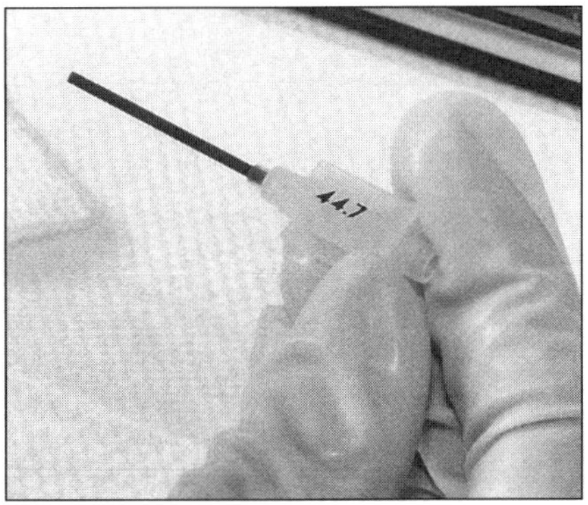

Figure 13-2a A pipette appropriately filled to its neck.

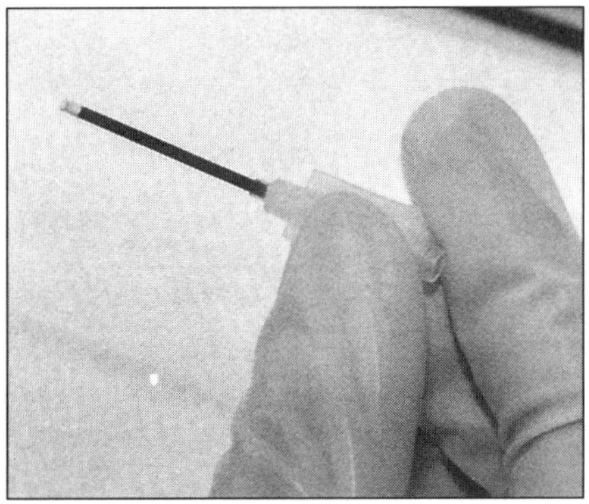

Figure 13-2b A pipette that is inappropriately underfilled.

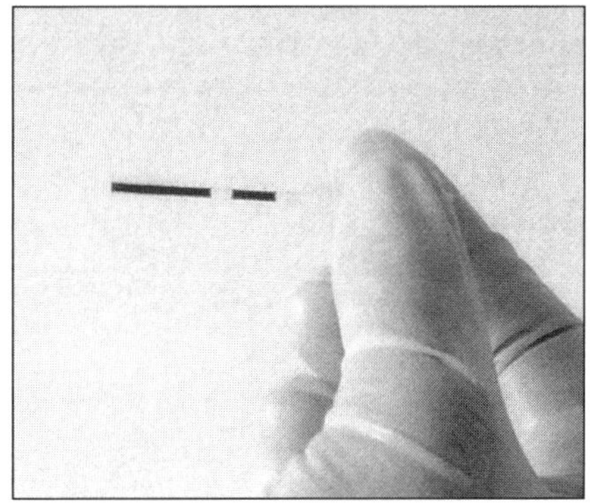

Figure 13-2c A pipette that contains an air bubble.

3. The outside of the pipette must be wiped off to remove excess blood, without removing blood from inside the pipette tip. If the blood from the outside of the pipette is introduced to the reservoir, it may affect the dilution.
4. Pipettes must be inserted into the reservoir without bumping the sides or ledges of the reservoir. If the pipette bumps the side or ledge of the reservoir, a drop of blood from inside the pipette may be removed.
5. To ensure that the pipette delivers an appropriate amount of blood into the reservoir, the following steps must be performed: 1) the reservoir must be squeezed tightly; 2) the index finger must be placed gently over the back of the pipette without pushing down on the back of the pipette (pushing down on the back of the pipette will force blood out of the tip of the pipette); 3) the pipette must be seated securely into the reservoir; 4) the finger should be removed from the back of the pipette; and 5) the reservoir should be released and then squeezed several times to rinse the pipette.

To ensure that the amount of diluent in the reservoir does not change, the following conditions must be met:

1. When squeezing the reservoir to rinse the pipette, care must be taken not to squeeze too hard, forcing the dilution out of the overflow chamber.
2. The bullet shield should be affixed to the top of the overflow chamber to prevent spills in the event that the Unopette® turns over during transport.

Preparing accurate dilutions at the collection site is sometimes difficult. Consequently, most facilities require that tests performed using the Unopette® system at the patient bedside be collected in a series. For example, a CBC collected by Unopette® would require preparing 3 dilutions at the patient's bedside.

Procedure 1:

Preparing Unopette® Dilutions from EDTA Samples

1. Wash hands. Don gloves and gown. Mix the EDTA sample well by inverting it several times. Unstopper the sample following the safety procedures for unstoppering specimens at your facility.
2. Select a Unopette® system. Place the reservoir on a flat surface, holding it securely with one hand. Using the other hand, pierce the diaphragm of the reservoir with the pointed end of the bullet shield (**Fig. 13-3**).
3. Remove the bullet shield from around the pipette.
4. Position the pipette so the overflow chamber rests between the index finger and thumb. The palm of the hand should be positioned underneath the pipette.
5. Position the tube of blood on an angle, so the blood approaches the rim of the tube.
6. Hold the pipette tip almost horizontal while touching the tip of the pipette to the blood in the EDTA tube (**Fig. 13-4**). The blood will displace the air in the pipette, and the tube will then fill with blood. Filling the pipette in this manner is called capillary action.

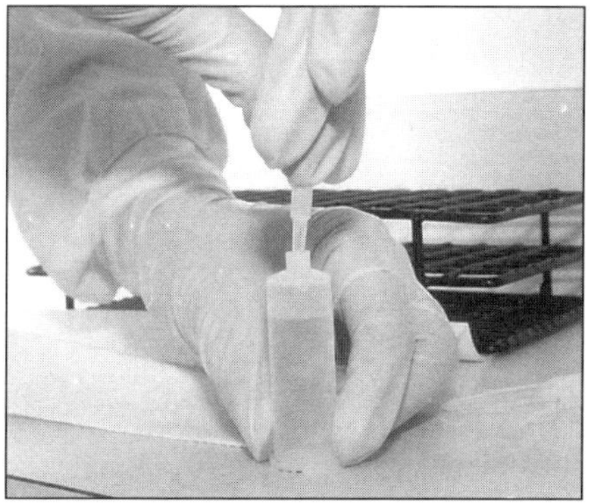

Figure 13-3 Pierce the diaphragm of the reservoir with the end of the bullet shield.

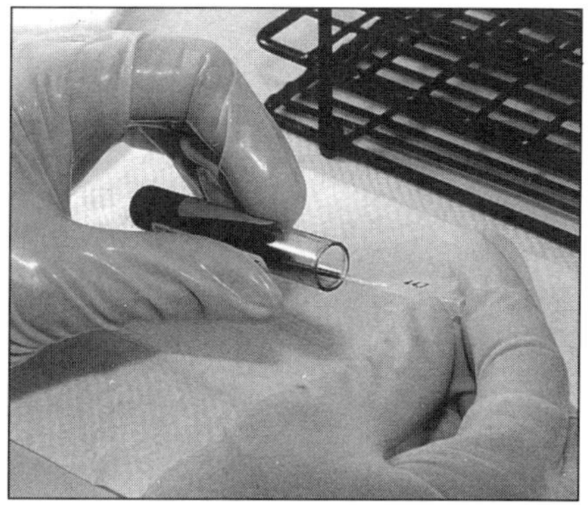

Figure 13-4 Touch the tip of the pipette to the blood in the tube.

7. Using a piece of gauze, wipe the excess blood from the outside of the pipette (**Fig. 13-5**). Be sure you do not draw blood out from the tip of the pipette by touching the tip of the pipette with the gauze. Touching the tip of the pipette with gauze will cause blood to be drawn out from the tip of the pipette.
8 Firmly squeeze the reservoir (**Fig. 13-6**).
9. Using the index finger, cover the overflow chamber of the pipette (**Fig. 13-7**). Be careful not to push down on the overflow chamber because this will force blood out of the tip of the pipette. Continue to squeeze the reservoir.
10. Secure the pipette onto the reservoir.

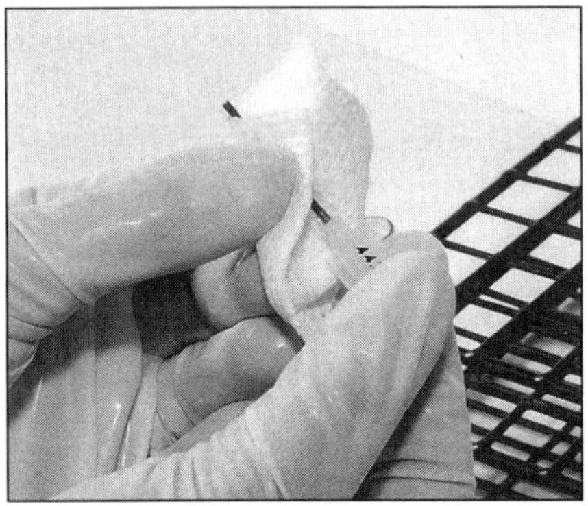

Figure 13-5 Wipe the excess blood from the outside of the pipette.

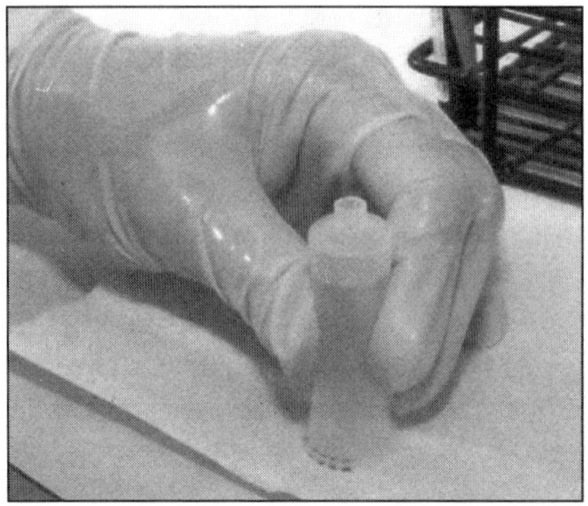

Figure 13-6 Firmly squeeze the reservoir.

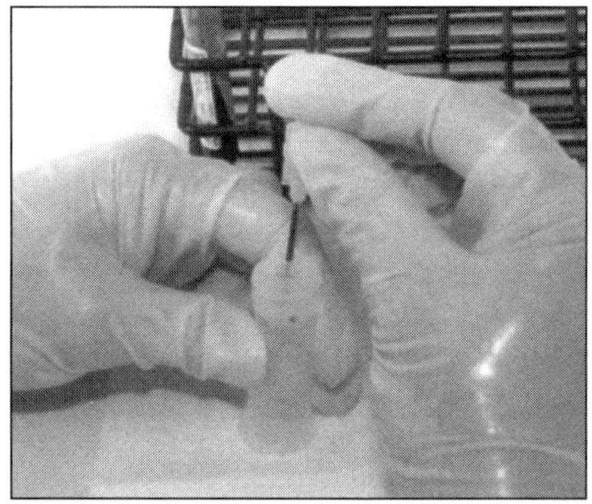

Figure 13-7 Cover the overflow chamber of the pipette with the index finger.

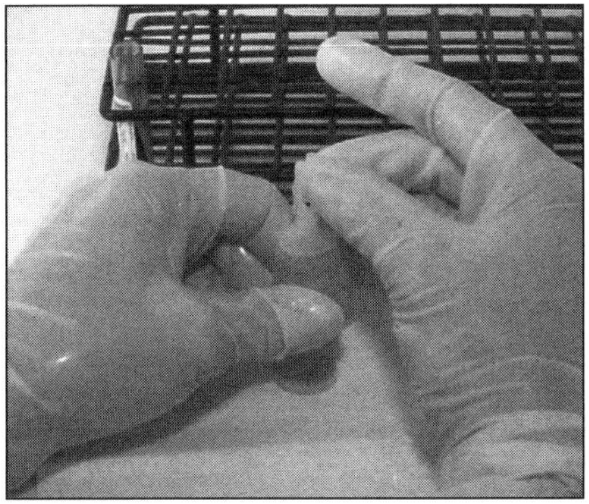

Figure 13-8 Remove the index finger from the overflow chamber.

11. Remove the index finger from the overflow chamber of the pipette (**Fig. 13-8**). Release the reservoir (**Fig. 13-9**). The negative pressure of the reservoir will draw the blood from the pipette into the diluent.
12. Squeeze the reservoir several times to rinse the pipette (**Fig. 13-10**). The dilution should be forced into, but not out of, the overflow chamber.
13. Place the bullet shield over the overflow chamber of the pipette (**Fig. 13-11**).
14. Invert the system several times to thoroughly mix the blood and diluent.
15. Prepare a label, incorporating all appropriate information (see Lab #10).
16. Repeat steps 1 through 15, using a second Unopette® system.
17. Remove gloves and protective clothing.
18. Wash hands.

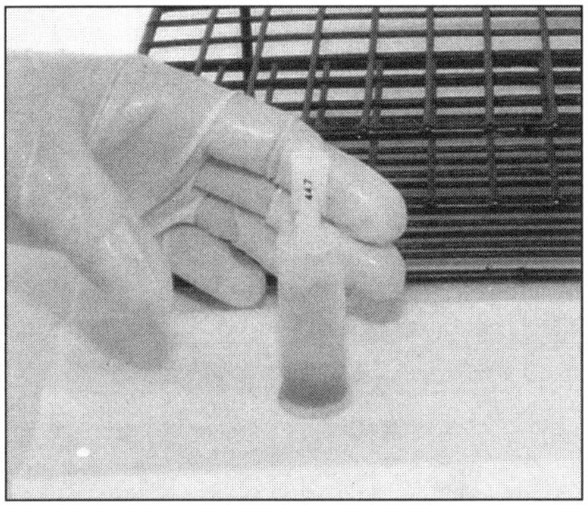

Figure 13-9 Release the reservoir.

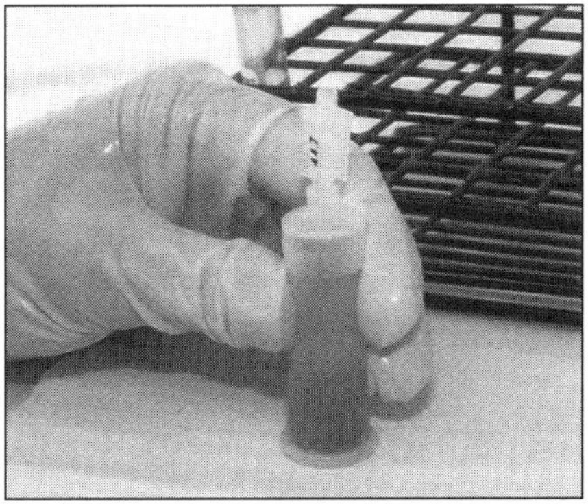

Figure 13-10 Squeeze the reservoir several times to rinse the pipette.

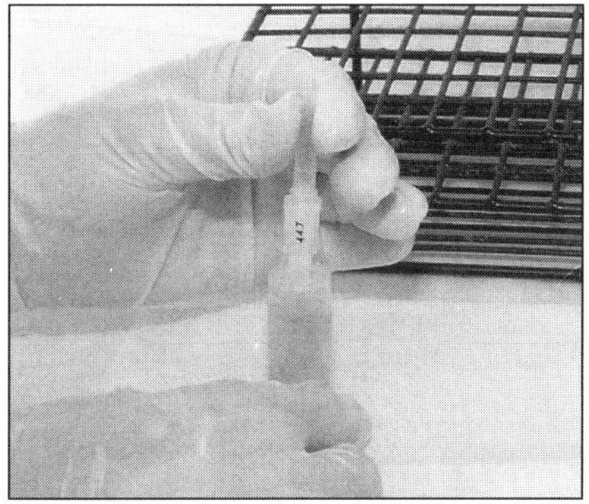

Figure 13-11 Place the bullet shield over the overflow chamber of the pipette.

Procedure 2: Preparing Unopette® Dilutions Following Skin Puncture

1. Wash hands. Don gloves and gown.
2. Choose 3 Unopette® Systems. Prepare each for dilution (steps 2 and 3 in Procedure 1).
3. Perform a skin puncture on your patient (see Lab #11).
4. Wipe off the first drop of blood.
5. Position the pipette as described in step 4 of Procedure 1.
6. Apply the tip of the pipette to the drop of blood at the skin puncture site. Be careful NOT to touch the wound with the pipette! Hold the pipette just below horizontal to the puncture site so it will fill by capillary action.
7. Once the pipette is appropriately filled, immediately prepare a dilution using the Unopette® System (steps 7 through 12 in Procedure 1).
8. Repeat steps 1 through 7, using the second and third Unopette® systems.
9. Provide appropriate postpuncture care for the patient (see Lab #11).
10. Place the bullet shield over the overflow chamber of the pipette.
11. Invert each system several times to thoroughly mix the sample and diluent.
12. Prepare a label for each dilution. Affix the label to the reservoir of each dilution.

Checklist:

Dilution Using EDTA Sample

Comments:

(A) Performed **(B) Needs Improvement** **(C) Not Performed**

_____ 1. Dons gloves, gown, and any other protective clothing required at your facility.
_____ 2. Appropriately mixes EDTA sample.
_____ 3. Removes stopper from EDTA tube following safety procedures established at your facility.
_____ 4. Places EDTA tube in test tube rack.
_____ 5. Punctures diaphragm of reservoir.
_____ 6. Tilts tube to fill pipette.
_____ 7. Fills pipette to appropriate level.
_____ 8. Fills pipette without introducing air bubbles.
_____ 9. Wipes off the outside of the pipette without withdrawing blood from the pipette tip.
_____ 10. Squeezes reservoir before inserting pipette.
_____ 11. Places finger over the back of the pipette without forcing blood out of the pipette tip.
_____ 12. Inserts pipette into reservoir without bumping the sides or ledges of the reservoir.
_____ 13. Seats pipette firmly into reservoir.
_____ 14. Releases finger from back of the pipette.
_____ 15. Releases reservoir.
_____ 16. Squeezes reservoir several times to rinse pipette.
_____ 17. Repeats steps 1 through 15 on second dilution.
_____ 18. Places bullet shield over pipette for transport.
_____ 19. Prepares label for reservoir, including all appropriate information.
_____ 20. Affixes label to reservoir.
_____ 21. Discards materials contaminated with blood in the biohazard bag.
_____ 22. Removes and discards gloves.
_____ 23. Washes hands.

Checklist: **(A) Performed** **(B) Needs Improvement** **(C) Not Performed**

Dilution After Skin Puncture

Comments:

_____ 1. Washes hands.
_____ 2. Dons gloves and gown.
_____ 3. Role play: Approaches patient. Explains procedure (if necessary).
_____ 4. Role play: Identifies patient, using 2-step method of patient identification.
_____ 5. Selects, prepares, and organizes equipment.
_____ 6. Selects site for skin puncture.
_____ 7. Applies warmer to site when appropriate.
_____ 8. Cleanses skin puncture site with alcohol.
_____ 9. Allows site to air dry.
_____ 10. Secures puncture site appropriately.
_____ 11. Punctures site with lancet at correct angle.
_____ 12. Wipes away first drop of blood.
_____ 13. Holds pipette horizontal to the puncture site to fill.
_____ 14. Fills pipette to the appropriate level.
_____ 15. Fills pipette without introducing air bubbles.
_____ 16. Wipes off the outside of the pipette without withdrawing blood from the pipette tip.
_____ 17. Squeezes reservoir before inserting pipette.
_____ 18. Places finger over the back of the pipette without forcing blood out of the pipette tip.
_____ 19. Inserts pipette into reservoir without bumping the sides or the edges of the reservoir.
_____ 20. Seats pipette firmly into reservoir.

Comments: **(A) Performed** **(B) Needs Improvement** **(C) Not Performed**

_____ 21. Releases finger from back of the pipette.
_____ 22. Releases reservoir.
_____ 23. Squeezes reservoir several times to rinse pipette.
_____ 24. Repeat steps 13 to 23 on the next 2 Unopettes®.
_____ 25. Provides appropriate postphlebotomy care to the patient.
_____ 26. Places bullet shields over pipettes.
_____ 27. Inverts Unopette® system several times to thoroughly mix specimen. Repeats on remaining 2 dilutions.
_____ 28. Prepares label for each dilution, including all appropriate information.
_____ 29. Affixes label to reservoir for each solution.
_____ 30. Discards lancet in needle disposal unit.
_____ 31. Discards materials contaminated with blood in the biohazard bag.
_____ 32. Removes equipment.
_____ 33. Removes gloves.
_____ 34. Washes hands.
_____ 35. Leaves patient courteously.

Study Questions
Lab 13

1. List at least 8 tests that may be collected using the Unopette® System.

2. Describe the Unopette® System used to collect each test listed in question #1.

3. A Unopette® System was used to collect a blood specimen by skin puncture for a CBC analysis. Would the phlebotomist be required to prepare a blood smear at the patient's bedside? Why or why not?

4. Are the capillary tubes used with the Unopette® System standardized? Explain.

5. What advantage(s) does the Unopette® System offer over other capillary blood collection systems?

6. Are there any disadvantages to using the Unopette® System?

LAB 14

Collection of Capillary Blood Using Large-Bore Capillary Tubes and Unopettes®

Objective

To gain expertise in performing skin puncture procedures; to properly collect blood specimens using large-bore capillary tubes and Unopette® system dilutions; to follow appropriate order of draw procedures when collecting multiple specimens by skin puncture

Equipment

70% isopropyl alcohol prep pads; Sterile gauze; Heel warmer; Blood lancet; Gloves; Gown; 3 large-bore capillary tubes; Capillary tube seals; 3 Unopette® systems for white blood cell and platelet determinations; 3 glass slides; 5 blank labels; Needle disposal unit; Biohazard bag

Order of Draw

Sometimes, specimens for several test procedures must be collected following skin puncture. When collecting blood specimens for multiple test procedures, the order of draw has important ramifications for the quality of specimen collected.

When collecting blood specimens by skin puncture, hematology specimens should be collected first. Platelet clumping is increased in blood specimens collected by skin puncture as compared to those collected by venipuncture. Consequently, to minimize the effects of platelet clumping on skin puncture samples, hematology studies must be collected first.

The Unopette® system used in this lab collects a sample for platelet and white blood cell determinations, which are hematology test procedures. Slides cannot be made from the dilution in the Unopette® system. Therefore, slides must be prepared with a drop of blood from the puncture site whenever hematology tests are collected using the Unopette® system. Blood collected for examination of cell morphology should be collected directly from the puncture site on clean microscopic slides. To prevent morphologic distortion, the blood should be wedge smeared and air dried immediately. The order of sample collection using the equipment selected for this lab is: 1) blood smear, 2) platelet count/white blood cell count (Unopette® system), and 3) large-bore capillary tubes.

Procedural Issues/Large-Bore Capillary Tubes

Large-bore capillary tubes are pencil-shaped tubes used to collect blood specimens following skin puncture. These tubes are larger in diameter and length than the tubes used for ABO typing and microhematocrit determinations. Large-bore capillary tubes are available in plain and heparinized types.

To obtain sufficient specimen for analysis, usually more than 1 large-bore capillary tube must be collected. The collection of a specimen in more than 1 tube is an advantage. For example, to perform a routine type and crossmatch analysis, at least 3 large-bore capillary tubes must be collected to supply the blood bank with sufficient specimen for analysis. If 1 of the tubes collected is

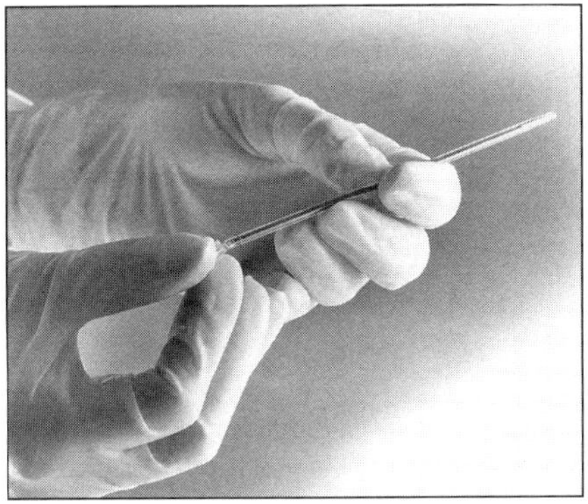

Figure 14-1 Insert nipple into the end of the tube.

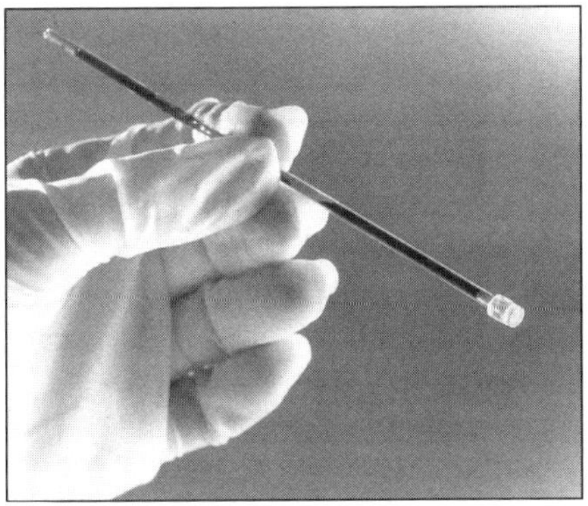

Figure 14-2 Properly sealed tube.

hemolyzed, there are 2 tubes remaining to perform the analysis. If the hemolyzed specimen was collected in 1 container, the entire specimen would have to be discarded and the patient redrawn.

To collect blood following skin puncture using large-bore capillary tubes, position the tube so the pointed end is toward the puncture site and the blunt end is away from the puncture site. Hold the tube between the thumb and index finger with the palm of the hand positioned underneath the tube. Squeeze the finger to form a drop of blood at the puncture site (refer to Lab #11). Touch the pointed end of the tube to the drop of blood. Be careful not to touch the wound! Hold the tube so the blunt end is just below horizontal to the drop of blood. The blood will run into the tube by capillary action. Continue to squeeze the finger until blood stops rolling into the tube. When this happens, release the finger, wait a brief second, and then squeeze again to repeat this procedure until specimen collection is completed.

If the blunt end of the large-bore capillary tube is held too far below horizontal, air bubbles may be introduced into the tube. Unlike the Unopette® system, air bubbles will not immediately compromise the quality of the sample unless they take up too much volume within the capillary tube. If too much volume within the tube is filled with air, the quantity of sample may be insufficient to perform the analysis requested. If a large-bore capillary tube contains air bubbles, the phlebotomist is well advised to collect an extra tube to ensure sufficient amount of sample for analysis.

To seal the large-bore capillary tube for transport, insert the nipple of the seal into the blunt end of the large-bore capillary tube (**Fig. 14-1**). Twist the cap to be sure it is securely affixed to the end of the tube (**Fig. 14-2**). Remove the stopper from a 10-mL red-top tube. Place the sealed large-bore capillary tubes into the unstoppered red-top tube. Label the red-top tube following standard procedures.

Procedure: Collection of Capillary Blood

1. Wash hands. Don gloves and gown.
2. Select, prepare, and organize the equipment.
3. Perform skin puncture (refer to Lab #11).
4. Collect sample. Prepare 2 blood smears first (refer to Lab #12). Prepare 3 Unopette® dilutions second (refer to Lab #13). Collect 3 large-bore capillary tubes last (refer to the Procedural Issues section of this lab).
5. Provide appropriate postpuncture care to the patient.
6. Label samples following standard labeling procedures.

Checklist: Collection of Capillary Blood

(A) Performed **(B) Needs Improvement** **(C) Not Performed**

Comments:

_____ 1. Washes hands.
_____ 2. Dons gloves and gown.
_____ 3. Role play: Approaches patient. Explains procedure.
_____ 4. Role play: Identifies patient, using 2-step method of patient identification.
_____ 5. Selects equipment.
_____ 6. Prepares Unopette® systems for dilution, prepares skin puncture equipment, and readies large-bore capillary tubes.
_____ 7. Organizes equipment.
_____ 8. Selects site for skin puncture.
_____ 9. Applies warmer to site when appropriate.
_____ 10. Cleanses skin puncture site with alcohol.
_____ 11. Allows site to air dry.
_____ 12. Secures puncture site appropriately.
_____ 13. Punctures site with lancet positioned at correct angle.
_____ 14. Wipes away the first drop of blood.
_____ 15. Places a drop of blood from the puncture site onto each of 2 slides by touching the slides to the drop of blood. Takes care not to touch the puncture site.

Comments: **(A) Performed** **(B) Needs Improvement** **(C) Not Performed**

_____ 16. Uses third slide as a spreader slide to prepare 2 blood smears.
_____ 17. Appropriately positions pipette (from the Unopette® System).
_____ 18. Fills pipette to the appropriate level.
_____ 19. Fills pipette without introducing air bubbles.
_____ 20. Wipes off the outside of the pipette without withdrawing blood from the pipette tip.
_____ 21. Squeezes reservoir before inserting pipette.
_____ 22. Places finger over the back of the pipette without forcing blood out of the pipette tip.
_____ 23. Inserts pipette into reservoir without bumping the sides or the edges of the reservoir.
_____ 24. Seats pipette firmly into reservoir.
_____ 25. Releases finger from back of the pipette.
_____ 26. Releases reservoir.
_____ 27. Squeezes reservoir several times to rinse pipette.
_____ 28. Repeats steps 14 through 27 on second and third Unopette® Systems.
_____ 29. Positions large-bore capillary tube so the pointed end touches the drop of blood.
_____ 30. Allows the tube to fill by capillary action.
_____ 31. Repeats steps 29 and 30 on the second and third large-bore capillary tubes.
_____ 32. Provides the patient with appropriate postpuncture care.
_____ 33. Places index finger over the overflow chamber of the Unopette® reservoir and inverts several times to mix the blood and diluent. Repeats on dilutions 2 and 3.
_____ 34. Places bullet shields over Unopette® pipettes for transport.

Comments: **(A) Performed** **(B) Needs Improvement** **(C) Not Performed**

_____ 35. Prepares labels and affixes to Unopette® reservoirs.
_____ 36. Places seals on the blunt end of large-bore capillary tubes.
_____ 37. Places sealed large-bore capillary tubes, sealed end down, in an unstoppered red-top tube.
_____ 38. Labels red-top tube following standard labeling procedures.
_____ 39. Removes equipment.
_____ 40. Discards lancet in needle disposal unit.
_____ 41. Discards materials contaminated with blood in the biohazard bag.
_____ 42. Appropriately discards other waste materials.
_____ 43. Inspects puncture site; applies bandage, if necessary.
_____ 44. Removes gloves and gown.
_____ 45. Washes hands.
_____ 46. Leaves patient courteously.

Checklist: Samples

Comments:

	Sample 1	Sample 2	Sample 3 (if indicated)	
Blood Smears				
1.	______	______	______	Has smooth, even surface.
2.	______	______	______	Has a thick portion, which tapers off into a thin portion.
3.	______	______	______	Ends in a feathered edge.
4.	______	______	______	Covers one half to two thirds of the slide.
5.	______	______	______	Has an appropriate thickness (is neither too thick nor too thin).
6.	______	______	______	Has a space on either side of the smear.
7.	______	______	______	Is appropriately labeled.
Unopette® Dilutions				
1.	______	______	______	No blood on the outside of the Unopette® system. (Blood on the outside of the Unopette® system may indicate spilling the dilution out of the overflow chamber.)
2.	______	______	______	No drops of blood on the lip or edges of the reservoir.
3.	______	______	______	Bullet shield positioned over the overflow chamber for transport.
4.	______	______	______	Appropriately labeled reservoir.
Large-Bore Capillary Tubes				
1.	______	______	______	Adequate sample.
2.	______	______	______	No air bubbles in sample.
3.	______	______	______	Properly sealed sample.
4.	______	______	______	Properly positioned sample for transport.
5.	______	______	______	No hemolysis of fluid component of sample.
6.	______	______	______	Properly labeled sample.

In reference to the sample checklist, were any sections marked "needs improvement"? ______________________________

What procedural errors resulted in the sections identified on the checklist?

____

Study Questions

Lab 14

1. List and describe at least 5 different types of lancets used for skin puncture.

____

____

2. What advantage(s) does each lancet in question #1 provide the phlebotomist and/or patient? ______________________________

____

3. What is the maximum appropriate lancet length for use on an infant? A 5-year-old child? An adult? ______________________________

____

____

4. List at least 2 reasons for performing skin puncture for blood collection instead of venipuncture. ______________________________

____

5. What is a Bard-Parker surgical blade? What is its relation to blood sample collection in the pediatric patient? ______________________________

____

LAB 15

Collection of Capillary Blood for Chemistry and Hematology Testing Using Capillary Blood Collection Tubes

Objective

To gain expertise in performing skin puncture procedures; to introduce the student to collection of capillary blood using a safety flow lancet and capillary blood collection tubes; to reinforce appropriate order of draw procedures; to reinforce quality control procedures as they relate to the collection of capillary blood specimens

Equipment

70% isopropyl alcohol prep pads; Sterile gauze; Heel warmer; Safety Flow Lancet; Gloves; Gowns; 1 red-top capillary blood collection tube; 1 lavender-top capillary blood collection tube; Needle disposal unit; Biohazard bag

Discussion

Supervisory personnel in the clinical laboratory select specific equipment to be used for the collection of capillary blood following skin puncture. The choice of capillary blood specimen collection containers is often based on the type of instrumentation used to perform the laboratory analyses.

Some facilities prefer capillary blood collection tubes instead of the large-bore capillary tubes and Unopette® systems described in Lab #14 for the collection of capillary blood samples. Blood specimens collected in capillary blood collection tubes offer 2 advantages to the medical technologist. First, blood specimens collected in capillary blood collection tubes may be directly incorporated into routine processing procedures. For example, blood smears may be prepared from the capillary blood collection tube in the laboratory, eliminating the preparation of blood smears at the patient's bedside. This characteristic offers the attractive advantage of convenience.

Second, the risk of percutaneous puncture to the medical technologist is significantly reduced when using capillary blood collection tubes instead of large-bore capillary tubes. After the specimen is accessioned, it is centrifuged. To access the fluid portion of the specimen (following centrifugation) collected in a large-bore capillary tube, the medical technologist must saw a ridge into the tube, using a tiny file. The tube is then snapped open at the ridge, and the fluid portion of the specimen removed for testing. Technologists and technicians can access the fluid portion of the capillary specimen collected in the capillary blood collection tube (following centrifugation) by removing the stopper and accessing the fluid portion of the specimen. The procedure does not involve sawing or breaking glass tubes. This offers the significant advantage of safety.

Safety Flow Lancet

The Safety Flow Lancet, like the blood lancet, is used once and discarded. The blade is encased in a plastic holder and is activated using a trigger mechanism. Following puncture, the blade is retracted into the plastic case, which is a

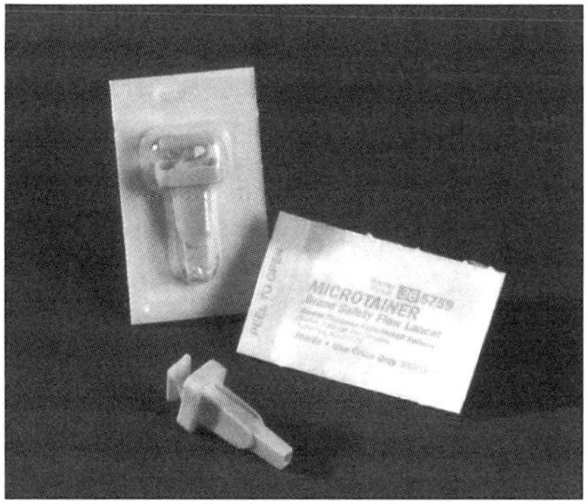

Figure 15-1 Safety Flow Lancets.

safety advantage. Safety Flow Lancets are available in a variety of lancet lengths (**Fig. 15-1**).

To use the Safety Flow Lancet, position the lancet between the thumb and middle finger. Place the index finger on the trigger mechanism. Position the Safety Flow Lancet on the skin puncture site selected so the widest part of the lancet intersects the fingerprints at a perpendicular angle. Using the thumb and middle finger, hold the Safety Flow Lancet firmly against the skin puncture site. Depress the trigger with the index finger. Do not pull the lancet away from the puncture site while depressing the trigger mechanism. This is a common error of beginners and may result in an inadequate puncture and an insufficient specimen.

Capillary Blood Collection Tubes

When collecting skin puncture blood samples with capillary blood collection tubes, hematology samples are collected first. It is not necessary to prepare slides at the patient's bedside, since the capillary blood collection tube will provide the hematology department with a whole blood sample suitable for the preparation of smears in the hematology laboratory.

After the chosen site has been prepared and punctured, wipe away the first drop of blood using a gauze pad. Apply pressure to the heel or finger to create a drop of blood at the puncture site. Allow the drop of blood to roll into the capillary blood collection tube through the flo-top opening. Blood flow from the puncture site is enhanced by holding the puncture site downward and gently applying continuous pressure to the surrounding tissue. Strong, repetitive pressure should not be applied, because this may cause hemolysis or contamination of the specimen with tissue fluid.

Whenever a sample is collected into an additive, the collection tube must be inverted at least 20 times following collection to ensure adequate mixing of sample with the additive. This is particularly true of samples collected by skin puncture into capillary blood collection tubes containing EDTA. If the skin puncture sample is not adequately mixed with the EDTA, the blood may clot before it arrives in the laboratory, rendering it useless for testing.

Quality Control

Whenever a blood specimen is collected after skin puncture, the following considerations must be addressed to provide the laboratory with a quality specimen for analysis. (Even though our practice of the procedure in this lab is limited to adults, capillary blood collection issues related to infants and pediatric patients will also be addressed.)

1. Standard patient identification procedures must always be followed.
2. Standard specimen labeling procedures must always be followed.
3. An infant's heel should not be punctured more than twice to collect a blood specimen.
4. A surgical blade should never be used to make a puncture in an infant's heel because the depth cannot be accurately and safely controlled.
5. The phlebotomist should be certain that the site is completely free of alcohol before making the puncture. If the specimen becomes contaminated with alcohol, the specimen will hemolyze.
6. Hematology specimens should be collected first, followed by chemistry and blood bank specimens. This order of draw for skin puncture specimens helps to reduce the amount of platelet clumping in capillary blood specimens.
7. If a collection into EDTA is slow or difficult, rotate the collector between drops to hasten the contact of blood to EDTA.
8. Excessive squeezing of the puncture site to secure a sample should be avoided to prevent hemolysis and contamination of the specimen with tissue fluid. This is best avoided by performing an adequate puncture.
9. Specimens collected by skin puncture should always be identified on the test requisition as "Skin Puncture Specimens."

Procedure:
Collection of Capillary Blood

1. Wash hands. Don gloves and gown.
2. Select, prepare, and organize equipment. To prepare equipment, peel back the paper from the lancet packaging. Do NOT remove the lancet! Place the opened package where the lancet will be easily attainable. Prepare the capillary blood collection tubes for collection by removing the color-coded stopper and replacing it with a Flo-Top collector, if necessary.
3. Perform skin puncture (refer to Lab #11, if necessary).
4. Collect sample as described using the EDTA capillary blood collection tube first. Tubes should be filled to a level between the lines.
5. Remove the Flo-Top collector, if necessary. Replace the color-coded stopper. Gently invert the tube at least 20 times.
6. Repeat steps 3 through 5, using the red-top tube.
7. Provide appropriate postpuncture care to the patient.
8. Label samples, following standard labeling procedures.
9. Discard lancet in needle disposal unit.
10. Dispose of waste materials in an appropriate manner.
11. Remove gloves and gown.
12. Wash hands.

Checklist:

Collection of Capillary Blood

Comments:

(A) Performed **(B) Needs Improvement** **(C) Not Performed**

_____ 1. Washes hands. Dons gloves and gown.
_____ 2. Role play: Approaches patient. Explains procedure (if necessary).
_____ 3. Role play: Identifies patient using 2-step method of patient identification.
_____ 4. Selects, prepares, and organizes equipment.
_____ 5. Selects site for skin puncture.
_____ 6. Applies warmer to site, when appropriate.
_____ 7. Cleanses skin puncture site with alcohol.
_____ 8. Allows site to air dry.
_____ 9. Secures puncture site appropriately.
_____ 10. Positions lancet perpendicular to fingerprints.
_____ 11. Depresses trigger, without lifting plastic case off the puncture site.
_____ 12. Wipes away the first drop of blood.
_____ 13. Squeezes finger to form drop of blood at puncture site.
_____ 14. Allows drop of blood to roll into the EDTA capillary blood collection tube through the flo-top.
_____ 15. Repeats steps 13 and 14 until the tube is full.
_____ 16. Caps the tube and inverts it 20 times to ensure mixing with EDTA.
_____ 17. Repeats steps 13 through 15 using the red-top evacuated tube.
_____ 18. Labels samples following standard labeling procedures.
_____ 19. Provides patient with appropriate postphlebotomy care.
_____ 20. Discards lancet in needle disposal unit.
_____ 21. Discards materials contaminated with blood in biohazard bag.
_____ 22. Appropriately discards other waste materials.
_____ 23. Removes equipment.
_____ 24. Inspects puncture site; applies bandage, if necessary.
_____ 25. Removes gloves. Washes hands.
_____ 26. Leaves patient courteously.

Checklist: Samples

(A) Performed **(B) Needs Improvement** **(C) Not Performed**

Comments:

	Sample 1	Sample 2	
1.	________	________	Adequate sample.
2.	________	________	Correct sequence of collection.
3.	________	________	Properly labeled sample.
4.	________	________	Properly mixed sample.
5.	________	________	Collected most of the specimen generated. (Did not "lose" sample as it ran down patient's finger.)
6.	________	________	Specimen was not hemolyzed.

In reference to the checklist, were any sections marked "needs improvement"?

____

What procedural errors resulted in the sections identified on the checklist?

____

What steps would you take to prevent the procedural errors identified above?

____

____

Study Questions
Lab 15

1. Compare and contrast at least 4 types of containers used for specimen collection following skin puncture. ______________________________

2. What advantage(s) does each device listed in question #1 offer over the other collection containers? ______________________________

3. What quantity of specimen can be obtained from a properly performed skin puncture? ______________________________

4. Why is it necessary to wipe away the first drop of blood following skin puncture? ______________________________

5. What step in the skin puncture procedure is MOST crucial in successfully obtaining a sufficient specimen for analysis? ______________________________

6. What factors may contribute to the hemolysis of a specimen following skin puncture? ______________________________

7. What is the maximum number of times an infant's heel should be punctured to successfully obtain a sample? ______________________________

LAB 16

Venipuncture

Objective

To introduce performing venipuncture on "patients";
to gain expertise in performing the venipuncture procedure

Equipment

Gown; Gloves; Tourniquet; 70% isopropyl alcohol prep pads; Dry gauze pads; Evacuated collection tubes; Holder; Needles; 1 syringe; Needle disposal unit; Biohazard bag

Discussion

For this lab, students will be required to perform venipuncture on "practice patients," who will be students from the class. In addition to acting as phlebotomists, students will be required to act as "practice patients." The Site Selection section of Lab #7 should be reviewed prior to initiating this exercise.

Anchoring the Vein

Successful venipuncture will rely to a large extent on how well the chosen vein is anchored. If a phlebotomist does not immobilize the vein adequately, the success of the procedure will depend on how well the surrounding musculature naturally anchors the vein. As a person ages, muscle tone decreases and skin loses its elasticity. Consequently, elderly patients rarely have veins sufficiently anchored by surrounding musculature and skin tissue to support needle insertion. Adequate anchoring of the veins selected as venipuncture sites on artificial arms is not as critical to the success of the procedure as anchoring veins selected as venipuncture sites on patients. Consequently, phlebotomists accustomed to performing venipuncture on artificial arms should be especially careful to anchor veins sufficiently in practice patients.

To adequately anchor a vein, place the index finger of your left hand (persons who are left-handed should use their right index finger) on the vein below the site selected. Place the middle finger of the left hand (persons who are left-handed should use their right middle finger) on the vein above the site selected. (Please note: Some phlebotomists prefer to use their thumb and index finger to anchor the vein. Other phlebotomists prefer to use one digit, either thumb or index finger, BELOW the puncture site to anchor the vein. Follow the recommendations of your instructor.) Gently push down on the vein selected, holding it in place until the needle has been inserted. If the thumb or index finger is removed before needle insertion, the vein will not be adequately anchored. This may lead to an unsuccessful venipuncture attempt. Once the bevel has entered the vein, the phlebotomist no longer needs to anchor the vein. The hand that was anchoring the vein may then be used to push the evacuated tube onto the needle.

Quality Control

To obtain a quality blood specimen for laboratory analysis, the following quality control procedures must be followed.

1. Proper patient identification is the most important step in securing a quality blood specimen. Proper patient identification involves the 2-step identification procedure (refer to Lab #6).
2. If a test procedure requires special preparation to be done by the patient, be sure to interview the patient prior to collecting the specimen to make sure that the instructions have been followed.
   For example, bleeding times are affected by aspirin ingestion. Consequently, patients should be interviewed prior to the procedure to determine whether they have taken any aspirin 7 to 10 days prior to the procedure.
   Some test procedures require a "fasting specimen." To secure a fasting specimen, the patient must not eat or drink anything after dinner the night before the test is to be collected except for water. Examples of tests requiring fasting specimens include glucose, triglycerides, cholesterol (certain procedures), total lipid profiles, chemistry profiles, and D-xylose.
3. Patients have the right to know the identity and professional status of every person providing them with service in the health care setting. Phlebotomists should always introduce themselves to the patient and state their intent. For example, the phlebotomist could approach the patient as follows: "Hello, my name is ______. I am from the laboratory, and I'm here to collect a blood specimen for a test your doctor has ordered. Have you ever had a blood specimen taken before?" Explain the procedure to be performed on the patient, if necessary. If the patient has questions about the purpose of the test or what the results will reveal, refer the patient to the physician.
4. Standard labeling procedures require the following information on each patient specimen: patient's full name; patient's hospital identification

Remember, the phlebotomist is the patients' "window" to the laboratory. Patients' perceptions of the quality of test results will be determined to a large degree by how they are addressed and treated by the phlebotomist.

number; patient's room and bed number; date and time of specimen collection; and phlebotomist's initials.

5. Be sure adequate amounts of sample are collected for the tests ordered. This is especially important when collecting blood specimens into additives, such as sodium citrate. Follow the guidelines at your facility for minimum acceptable volumes.

6. Be sure tests are collected in appropriate containers. Every facility provides its staff with a procedure book, which details specimen requirements for each test procedure. If you are not sure about what tube to draw, consult the procedure manual. If an inappropriate tube is accidentally collected, the specimen must be redrawn, using the correct tube. DO NOT POUR THE CONTENTS OF ONE TUBE INTO ANOTHER!

7. Specimens should be transported to the lab in a timely fashion.

8. The tourniquet should not be left on the patient's arm for longer than 1 minute. A tourniquet left on too long may cause hemoconcentration and inaccurate test results.

9. The following sites are inappropriate for venipuncture: above an IV; arm on the side a mastectomy was performed; edematous areas; hematomas; arm in which blood is being transfused; areas that are extensively scarred; and arms in which cannulas, fistulas, or vascular grafts have been placed.

10. Tubes containing additives should be gently inverted 5 to 10 times following venipuncture to mix the blood specimen with anticoagulant or additive.

11. When multiple specimens are collected from a patient at one time, the appropriate order of draw is as follows: 1) blood cultures; 2) red or SST evacuated tubes; 3) coagulation tubes (blue stopper) (a blue-stoppered evacuated tube intended for a coagulation test should never be drawn first, because the thromboplastin from the site of the venipuncture may invalidate coagulation results. If the blue-stoppered tube is the only tube to be drawn, it should be preceded by a red-stoppered "discard" tube); 4) heparinized evacuated tubes (green stopper); 5) EDTA evacuated tubes (lavender stopper); and 6) sodium fluoride/potassium oxalate evacuated tubes (gray stopper).

12. The number of blood collection attempts on any patient should be limited to 2.

Performing Venipuncture on Fellow Students

Prior to this lab, students have had limited experience performing invasive procedures on each other. Performing venipuncture on a fellow student may be stressful for the practicing phlebotomist, not to mention the practice patient. To help reduce the anxiety associated with performing venipuncture on a fellow student, it is recommended that students focus their attention on the arm, from the shoulder to the wrist, and mentally dissociate the arm from the rest of the person.

Performing the "Painless" Venipuncture

Phlebotomists are always concerned about the possibility of hurting their patients. The following suggestions may help to make venipuncture as painless as possible:

1. For the greatest chance of securing a blood specimen, choose the widest, deepest part of the vein for a venipuncture site. This choice is determined while palpating the vein. Be very specific about site selection. Remember, missing the site selected (with the needle) by as little distance as a millimeter can mean the difference between success and failure in obtaining a sample (**Fig. 16-1**).

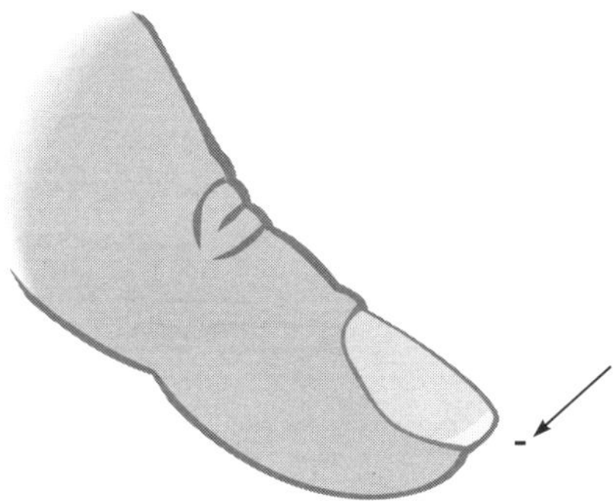

Figure 16-1 The length of a millimeter as compared to a thumb.

2. When choosing a site for venipuncture, look for "markers" to help identify the site. For example, while palpating the vein, you identify the widest, deepest part of the vein as being "a hair past that freckle." The needle should be inserted in that EXACT SPOT and in the SAME DIRECTION as the vein.

3. To ensure a successful venipuncture, the vein must be anchored before inserting the needle. If the vein is not sufficiently anchored, the needle will merely push the vein aside instead of piercing the vessel wall. The

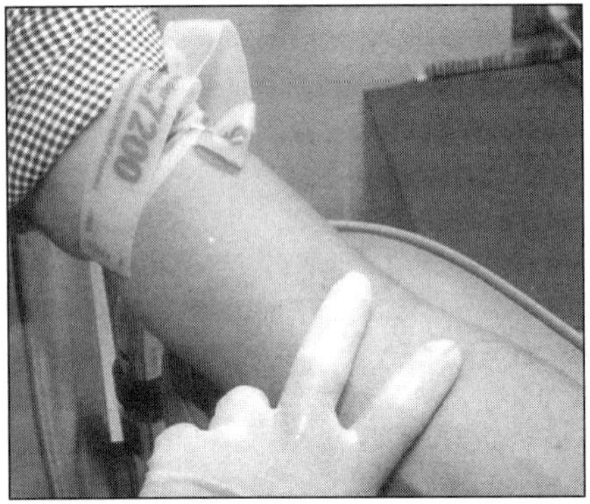

Figure 16-2 Anchoring technique using the index and middle fingers.

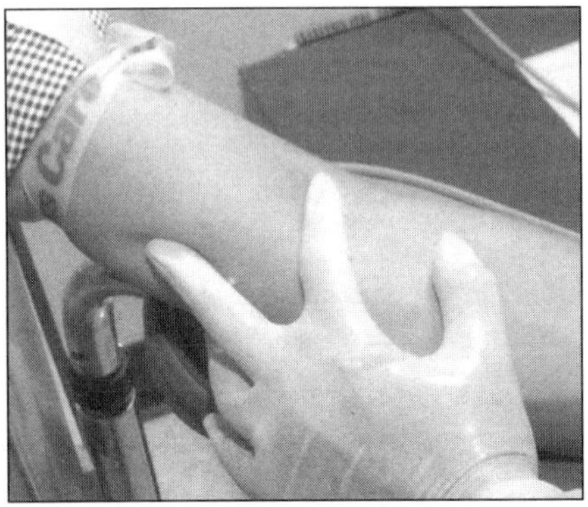

Figure 16-3 Anchoring technique using the thumb and index finger.

phlebotomist should use the index finger and middle finger or thumb and index finger to hold the vein stationary until the needle has pierced the vessel wall (**Fig. 16-2**, **Fig. 16-3**).

4. The phlebotomist should try to correlate the location of the deepest, widest part of the vein with how deep the bevel of the needle must be inserted to reach that part of the vein. The bevel of the needle should be inserted in one motion and stopped when the phlebotomist perceives the needle has reached the point selected. Many times, while piercing a vessel wall, the phlebotomist can feel some resistance on the needle. Once the vessel wall has been pierced, the resistance on the needle no longer can be felt. At this point, the insertion of the needle should stop.
5. When pushing tubes onto the needle or removing tubes from the back of the needle keep the holder ABSOLUTELY STILL. To accomplish this, rest the knuckles of the hand positioning the holder on the patient's arm to help keep the holder securely in position. In addition, focus attention on the point at which the needle is inserted into the arm. If the holder is not steady, the needle will move. If the needle is moving, adjustments must be made to keep the holder still.
6. Be careful not to pull the holder back in an attempt to ease the tube onto the back of the holder.
7. When changing tubes, sometimes it is easier to pull the tube off the back of the needle, if the holder is used for leverage. This is only appropriate, however, if the holder remains stationary.
8. Once the needle is positioned properly and blood is being collected in an evacuated tube, continue to position the needle forward and downward. New phlebotomists sometimes unwittingly pull up on the needle underneath the skin or slowly pull back on the needle while the tube is filling. Either case will result in the needle coming out of the vein, resulting in an unsuccessful venipuncture and more patient discomfort. To be sure the needle is held

The number of blood collection attempts by a phlebotomist should be limited to 2. If, after 2 attempts, the student or phlebotomist has not secured an acceptable blood specimen, the supervisor should be notified.

downward and forward, the phlebotomist should concentrate on the site of entry in the arm. Once again, if the holder is being moved, it will be indicated by the needle being moved at the site of entry. The phlebotomist should focus on the point of entry and only glance down at the tube to determine whether or not it is filled.

9. When withdrawing the needle, do NOT push down on the gauze to apply pressure to the puncture site until after the needle is withdrawn. Pushing down on the needle while withdrawing it may push the point of the needle through the vessel wall on the back of the vessel, and this can be very painful. Do not apply pressure until the needle is entirely removed from the patient's arm.

If No Blood Appears in the Tube Following Venipuncture

On occasion, once the evacuated tube has been pushed onto the back of the needle, no blood appears in the tube. If this is the case, the phlebotomist must evaluate the situation to make an adjustment with the needle.

1. Pull the needle back a small distance (not to exceed the length of the bevel). If blood still does not appear in the tube, advance the needle a little deeper (not to exceed the length of the bevel). The direction the needle should be moved first is determined by the phlebotomist. The phlebotomist must evaluate the position of the vein, relative to the bevel of the needle. The adjustment made with the needle (ie, moving it in deeper or pulling it back) is based on this evaluation. This adjustment is appropriate if the needle is positioned directly over the vein. The causes of this problem include not pushing the needle in deep enough, pushing the needle in too deep (ie, through the vein), or holding the bevel against the vein wall.

2. Sometimes, the needle ends up next to the vein. This usually occurs if the vein has not been anchored well or if the phlebotomist does not insert the needle exactly in the site selected. (Remember, missing the site selected by a millimeter can result in missing the vein.) In this event, the phlebotomist should: repalpate the vein; determine the location of the vein relative to the bevel of the needle (which can be accomplished by repalpating the vein); reanchor the vein; pull back on the needle, being careful not to expose the bevel; and redirect the needle and insert it into the side of the vein.

3. If the phlebotomist is reasonably sure that the needle is in the vein, another evacuated tube of the same stopper color can be substituted. On occasion, evacuated tubes lose their vacuum. Substituting another tube for the original one may correct this situation.
4. Sometimes untying the tourniquet will cause blood to begin to enter the tube. This is most often true if the tourniquet was tied too tightly.
5. If you have attempted these 4 steps and no blood appears in the tube, release the tourniquet, remove the tube from the back of the needle, withdraw the needle, and provide routine postphlebotomy care to the patient. Inform the patient that you were unsuccessful and ask if you may try to perform the venipuncture again. If you have already made 2 attempts, inform the patient that someone else will be back to attempt the venipuncture. Remember, remain calm and courteous.
6. Sometimes the needle will become dislodged from the evacuated tube holder while the needle is in the patient's arm. The appropriate course of action is to untie the tourniquet and remove the needle from the patient's arm. Exercise extreme caution to prevent accidental self-puncture with the contaminated needle.

Causes of Hemolysis

One of the most common reasons for specimen rejection in the clinical laboratory is hemolysis of the specimen. Hemolysis is the rupturing or destruction of red blood cells. When red blood cells are ruptured or destroyed, hemoglobin is liberated into the fluid portion of the blood. This fluid portion of the blood is called plasma if the blood has been collected into an anticoagulant, or serum if the blood has been allowed to clot. The normal color of plasma or serum is yellow. When hemoglobin is liberated into the fluid portion of the blood, the fluid may become pink or red.

Hemolysis can be detected in blood specimens as a result of certain clinical conditions. Clinical conditions characterized by hemolysis include hemolytic anemia, liver disease, and transfusion reactions. A more common cause of specimen hemolysis, however, is inappropriate specimen collection technique. Following are some collection errors that may result in hemolysis of the specimen.

- Using a needle that is too small for the force of the vacuum of the tube
- Shaking an additive tube too forcefully, instead of gently inverting it
- Drawing blood from a hematoma
- Centrifuging blood specimens before they have been allowed to clot completely
- Securing the specimen as a result of a traumatic venipuncture

Hemolyzed specimens interfere with certain analyses. To the right are examples of test procedures affected by hemolysis.

Chemistry Tests

Acid phosphatase
Alanine aminotransferase
Albumin
Aldolase
Alkaline phosphatase
Aspartate aminotransferase
Bilirubin
Chemistry profile tests
Chloride
Cholesterol
Creatine phosphokinase
Haptoglobin
Iron
Lactic dehydrogenase
Lipase
Magnesium
Phosphate
Phosphorous
Plasma hemoglobin
Potassium
Protein

Hematology Tests

Complete blood cell count
Hemoglobin

Blood Bank Tests

Antibody screens
Compatibility tests (Crossmatches)
RhoGAM work-ups

Immunology Tests

ASO titers
Cold agglutinin titers

Coagulation Tests

APTT
PT

Procedure: Venipuncture

1. Consult the record sheet to determine what test must be collected. Wash hands. Don gloves and gown.
2. Role play: Approach patient.
3. Role play: Identify the patient.
4. Role play: Explain procedure to the patient. Interview the patient concerning patient preparation guidelines if appropriate.
5. Select, prepare, and organize equipment (refer to Lab #11, if necessary).
6. Secure tourniquet.
7. Select a venipuncture site by palpating for a vein.
8. Release the tourniquet.
9. Cleanse the site with 70% alcohol. Begin at the puncture site and move the alcohol pad outward in concentric circles.
10. Allow the site to air dry.
11. Reapply the tourniquet. Take care that the ends of the tourniquet do not touch the cleansed venipuncture site.
12. Position the holder between your thumb and index finger (refer to Lab #10).
13. Uncap the needle. Inspect the needle for manufacturing defects.
14. Anchor the vein selected using an appropriate technique.
15. Position the needle appropriately (refer to Lab #10).
16. Insert the needle bevel up.
17. Push the evacuated tube onto the back of the needle (refer to Lab #10).
18. Keep the holder absolutely still. If blood does not enter the tube, or if blood starts to enter the tube and then stops, the position of the needle may be adjusted by moving the holder. However, these circumstances are the ONLY appropriate times to move the needle once it has entered the vein.
19. Allow the tube to fill.
20. Keeping the holder still, pull the evacuated tube off the back of the needle. A second tube may be pushed onto the back of the needle and allowed to fill.

21. Once blood begins to enter the second tube, release the tourniquet within 1 minute of application.
22. Pull the evacuated tube off the back of the holder. Allow it to rest in the holder.
23. Place a piece of gauze over the puncture site.
24. Withdraw the needle.
25. Role play: Instruct the patient to apply pressure to the puncture site.
26. Remove the evacuated tube from the holder and place the needle into a needle disposal unit.
27. If the evacuated tube(s) contains an additive, invert gently several times to mix the blood with the additive.
28. Label the tubes collected immediately following collection.
29. Inspect the puncture site. Provide appropriate postphlebotomy care.
30. Record the specimen on the Venipuncture Record Sheet. Fill in the appropriate information. Allow the instructor to initial the record sheet.

Checklist: Venipuncture

(A) Performed **(B) Needs Improvement** **(C) Not Performed**

Comments:

_____ 1. Washes hands. Dons gloves and gown.
_____ 2. Role play: Approaches patient.
_____ 3. Role play: Identifies patient.
_____ 4. Role play: Explains procedure. Interviews patient.
_____ 5. Selects, prepares, and organizes equipment.
_____ 6. Secures tourniquet.
_____ 7. Selects venipuncture site.
_____ 8. Releases the tourniquet.
_____ 9. Cleanses the site with 70% alcohol.
_____ 10. Allows the site to air dry.
_____ 11. Reapplies the tourniquet.
_____ 12. Positions the holder between thumb and index finger.
_____ 13. Uncaps the needle. Inspects the needle for manufacturing defects.
_____ 14. Anchors the vein selected.
_____ 15. Positions the needle at the appropriate angle and in the appropriate direction.
_____ 16. Inserts the needle bevel up.
_____ 17. Pushes the evacuated tube onto the back of the needle, keeping the holder absolutely still.
_____ 18. Draws evacuated tubes in the appropriate order.
_____ 19. Appropriately (within 1 minute of application) releases tourniquet.
_____ 20. Pulls the evacuated tube off the back of the needle and allows it to rest in the holder.
_____ 21. Places a piece of gauze over the puncture site.
_____ 22. Withdraws the needle. Instructs patient to apply pressure to the site.

Comments: **(A) Performed** **(B) Needs Improvement** **(C) Not Performed**

______ 23. Removes the evacuated tube from the holder and places the needle into a needle disposal unit.
______ 24. Inverts tube gently several times to mix the blood with the additive.
______ 25. Labels the tubes appropriately.
______ 26. Records the specimen on the venipuncture record sheet.
______ 27. Discards materials contaminated with blood into the biohazard bag.
______ 28. Appropriately discards other waste materials.
______ 29. Inspects puncture site; applies bandage, if needed.
______ 30. Removes all equipment.
______ 31. Washes hands.
______ 32. Leaves patient courteously.

Record Sheet: Single Draws

Instructions: Students must complete a minimum of 25 venipunctures to successfully complete the lab. Some of the venipunctures listed below correspond to venipunctures assigned in subsequent labs. Tests to be collected have been identified under the "Tests Ordered" column. To begin, the student should consult the venipuncture record sheet for the test ordered. The student should select the appropriate evacuated tube and other necessary equipment. After completing the venipuncture, the student should record the patient's name under the "Patient" column and fill in the remainder of the chart. The student should present the labeled specimen and completed record sheet to the instructor. If the specimen is acceptable, and if the information on the venipuncture record chart is correct, the instructor will initial the venipuncture record sheet under the column marked "Instructor's Initials." It is recommended that students complete the record sheet in the order established. That is, collect specimen 1 first, 2 second, and so on, until the record is completed.

No.	Instructor's Initials	Patient's Name	Tests Ordered	Stopper Color(s)	Tube Additive	Department	Clinical Significance
1	______	______	CBC	______	______	______	______
2	______	______	Hemoglobin	______	______	______	______
3	______	______	Hematocrit	______	______	______	______
4	______	______	ALAT	______	______	______	______
5	______	______	LDH isoenzymes	______	______	______	______
6	______	______	CK isoenzymes	______	______	______	______
7	______	______	Lipase	______	______	______	______

No.	Instructor's Initials	Patient's Name	Tests Ordered	Stopper Color(s)	Tube Additive	Department	Clinical Significance
8			Creatinine				
9			Bilirubin				
10			RhoGAM work-up				
11			T3, T4, T7				
12			HBsAg				
13			Blood culture				
14			Cold agglutinin				
15			Type and crossmatch				
16			Fibrinogen				
17			Carotene				
18			Sickle cell screen				
19			FTA				

Record Sheet: Multidraws

No.	Instructor's Initials	Patient's Name	Tests Ordered	Stopper Color(s)	Tube Additive	Department	Clinical Significance
1			Gentamicin				
			Prothrombin time				
2*			Cholesterol				
			APTT				
3*			Glucose				
			LE Prep				
4			ANA				
			Cortisol				
5			Digoxin				
			FDP				
6*			Chem profile				
			CBC				

* Tests requiring special patient preparation.

Study Questions

Lab 16

Listed below are the stopper colors of several evacuated tubes. For each tube:

A. Identify the type of specimen usually collected in that stopper color tube

B. Identify the additive

C. Identify the action of the additive on the blood specimen

D. Identify a characteristic of the additive that makes it MOST appropriate for the specimen being collected

The first one is completed as an example.

Gray

A. Glucose

B. Sodium fluoride and potassium oxalate

C. Precipitates calcium

D. Acts as a glycolytic inhibitor

1. Lavender

A. ______________________________

B. ______________________________

C. ______________________________

D. ______________________________

2. Red and Gray

A. ______________________________

B. ______________________________

C. ______________________________

D. ______________________________

3. Blue

A. ______________________________

B. ______________________________

C. ______________________________

D. ______________________________

LAB 17

Blood Cultures

Objective

To introduce the collection procedure for blood culture specimens

Equipment

Gloves; Gown; Tourniquet; Blood culture prep kit; Sterile gauze; Holder; 3 needles; 3 evacuated tubes containing SPS (yellow-top tubes); Needle disposal unit; Biohazard bag

Discussion

Blood cultures are among the most important cultures performed by the clinical microbiology department. Blood cultures are used by physicians to rule out or confirm septicemia and/or bacteremia. Septicemia and bacteremia infections may be severe and potentially life threatening.

Blood culture analysis is usually ordered before the initiation of antimicrobial therapy, usually in a series (eg, 3x). Blood culture collection is often timed to be performed just before the patient's next expected temperature rise. Bacteremia, the presence of bacteria in the blood, may be transient, intermittent, or continuous. By collecting blood specimens in a series, the likelihood of detecting the causative organism in any of these situations is increased. If a physician suspects the bacteremia to be the result of a localized infection, the entire series may be ordered to be collected at once. In this instance, it is appropriate for the phlebotomist to collect specimens for blood culture analysis from 3 different sites.

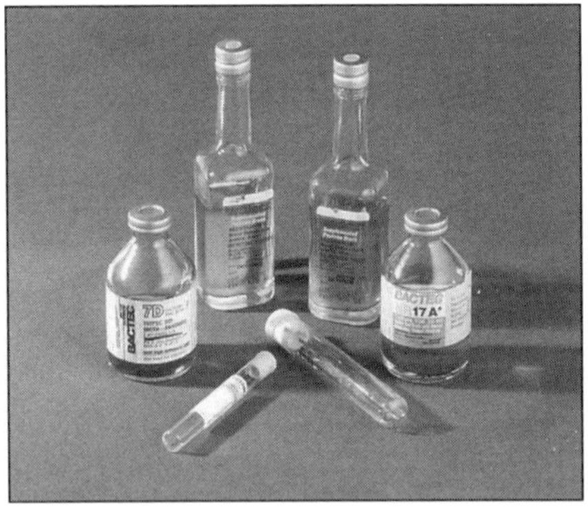

Figure 17-1 Blood culture specimen bottles.

Blood cultures indicate the severity of an infection and identify the causative organism. The procedure also determines the antimicrobial susceptibility of the causative organism. Normal values are negative for growth. Normally, no organisms of any kind should be present in the patient's bloodstream.

Various types of blood culture specimen collection containers are on the market. Some are used with the standard evacuated blood collection system. Others employ a syringe to inoculate blood culture bottles (**Fig. 17-1**). Utilization procedures for all of the commercially prepared collection containers require an aseptic technique. If multiple samples are collected, the blood culture specimen is always collected first.

Site Selection

Blood culture site selection should follow the same basic guidelines as for routine venipunctures. In the clinical setting, blood cultures are usually ordered in a series (eg, 3x). Site selection will also be influenced by the sample number in the series of cultures ordered by a patient's physician. The primary blood culture specimen should be obtained from 2 separate sites. Subsequent blood culture specimens should be obtained from alternate sites. Blood specimen collections from the artificial arms should be approached as if the 2 assigned draws were the first 2 collected in a series of 3.

Site Preparation

Blood normally is sterile. That is, blood normally does not contain bacteria or other organisms. Bacteria do normally exist on the skin surface. It is imperative (for quality test results) NOT to introduce bacteria into the specimen being collected. Before the collection of a specimen for blood culture analysis, the selected venipuncture site must be prepared by aseptic technique. An example of aseptic technique is outlined in the procedure below.

Once the site has been prepared DO NOT REPALPATE! Repalpating the site may contaminate it. The only exceptions to this rule are: 1) if the phlebotomist has appropriately cleansed the gloved finger to be used to repalpate; or 2) if the phlebotomist is using sterile gloves and has not contaminated the finger to be used to repalpate the venipuncture site.

Labeling

When labeling blood culture specimens, routine labeling procedures should be followed. In addition, the label should include the site used for collection and the number of the sample in the collection series (eg, R arm, 2nd of 3). Sites are varied throughout the series of blood culture collection to increase the rate of recovering pathogenic bacteria. Consequently, the blood culture specimens should be labeled with the collection site and the sequence in the collection series as a point of reference for the subsequent draw. In addition, the site of collection and the sequence in the collection series may impact the interpretation of the results. Therefore, the information must be available to the technologist and the attending physician.

Proper skin antisepsis prior to venipuncture is critical for quality blood culture results. Since blood is normally sterile, the recovery of any microorganisms in the blood culture specimen requires further investigation. If a physician receives a report identifying a microorganism recovered from a blood culture specimen, the information must be evaluated within the context of the patient's condition.

Quality Control

If a blood culture specimen was collected from an improperly prepared site, the specimen may be contaminated with microbial flora of the skin. A positive blood culture that is the result of collection error—and NOT due to pathogens in the patient's bloodstream—is referred to as a "false positive." Contamination of blood culture specimens should be limited to less than 3% (ie, less than 3 out of every 100 positive blood cultures should be the result of contamination during the blood collection procedure). If the microbiology department determines that the contamination rate exceeds 3%, it will investigate. The phlebotomists who collected the contaminated cultures will be identified, and their technique will be evaluated and, if necessary, modified.

If the microorganism recovered is recognized as a common skin contaminant (eg, *Staphylococcus epidermidis* or *Corynebacterium*), one might think it could be safely ruled out as the causative organism of the patient's bacteremia. However, in certain conditions, such as infective endocarditis (especially in prosthetic heart valves), the causative organism may be one of the microorganisms commonly referred to as "skin contaminants." Therefore, the preparation of the venipuncture site prior to the collection of a specimen for blood culture analysis must be meticulously performed to reduce the contamination of blood culture specimens with microbial flora of the skin.

To accomplish this, the phlebotomist should: 1) use appropriate cleansing agents; 2) apply the cleansing agents in the appropriate order; and 3) NEVER repalpate the site after it was cleansed by aseptic technique. It is only appropriate to repalpate if the gloved finger to be used was cleansed appropriately or if sterile gloves are used.

When blood cultures are ordered as part of multiple specimen collections, blood culture specimens are always collected first. The needles used for blood specimen collection are, of course, sterile. If an evacuated tube is used prior to the blood culture specimen collection, the needle will become contaminated, and microorganisms will be introduced into the specimen tube, possibly resulting in a false-positive result. Collection sequence following the blood culture is the same as for routine venipuncture procedures.

Volume of specimen collected is critical to the validity of test results. Too little blood may result in a false-negative test result. Failure to recover organisms present in a blood culture specimen is a "false negative." Excessive blood may clot in the collection tube, rendering recovery of microorganisms difficult or impossible.

False-negative specimens may occur if the specimen is contaminated with iodine. Iodine contamination is usually the result of excess iodine on the stopper prior to inoculation. False-negative results may also occur in the Bactec® blood culture specimen collection system if air is injected into the anaerobic culture bottle.

Procedure: Aseptic Technique

1. Follow routine procedures for handwashing, gloving, gowning, equipment preparation and organization, patient approach, patient identification, and venipuncture site selection (refer to Labs #10 and #16).
2. Explain to patients that their physician has ordered a series of tests requiring a series of venipunctures. Explain that the venipuncture procedure will be performed several times over a particular time span.
3. Loosen tourniquet.
4. Remove the alcohol/acetone scrub from the prep kit. Squeeze the handle to break the ampule contained within the prep kit.
5. Continue to squeeze the broken ampule until the sponge becomes saturated.
6. Cleanse the site, moving the alcohol/acetone scrub back and forth across the venipuncture site for 60 seconds.

7. Remove the ampule containing the iodine from the scrub kit. Break the ampule by squeezing it in the middle.
8. Continue to squeeze the ampule until the cotton at the end is completely saturated with iodine.
9. Position the iodine over the puncture site. Squeeze the ampule to apply iodine to the puncture site.
10. Move the iodine ampule in concentric circles outward.
11. Using the iodine ampule, paint the top of the collection container.
12. Allow the site and the top of the collection container to air dry.
13. Reapply the tourniquet. Be careful the ends of the tourniquet do not fall onto the puncture site, thereby contaminating it. (If the tourniquet does accidentally touch the prepared puncture site, the site must be recleansed.)
14. Perform the venipuncture, following routine venipuncture procedures. Do not repalpate! If you must repalpate the site, follow the guidelines listed under the Site Preparation section of this lab.
15. If the blood culture is one of a series of samples to be drawn from a patient, the blood culture must be collected first.
16. Provide appropriate postphlebotomy care to the patient.
17. Label the blood specimen collected, following standard labeling procedures. Be sure to include the site used and the number of the specimen in the series ordered.
18. Discard waste materials following standard procedures.
19. Record the draw (#13) on the Venipuncture Record Sheet (Lab #16).

Assignment

1. Collect 2 specimens from the artificial arms for blood culture analysis.
2. Have your lab partner observe the blood culture specimen collections from the artificial arms.
3. Your lab partner must complete a checklist for each blood culture specimen collection from the artificial arms.
4. Label the specimens collected from the artificial arm. (Assume the 2 draws are the first draws in a series of 3.)
5. Present the labeled specimen tubes and checklists to your instructor.
6. After completing specimen collection for blood culture analysis on the artificial arms to the satisfaction of the instructor, collect a blood specimen for blood culture analysis from your lab partner. Label the specimen. (Assume the specimen is the second collected in a series of 3.) Record the specimen in the appropriate place on the Venipuncture Record Sheet.

Checklist:

Venipuncture of Artificial Arms for Blood Culture Specimen Collection #1

Comments:

(A) Performed **(B) Needs Improvement** **(C) Not Performed**

_____ 1. Washes hands. Dons gloves and gown.
_____ 2. Role play: Approaches patient.
_____ 3. Role play: Identifies patient.
_____ 4. Role play: Explains procedure to the patient.
_____ 5. Selects, prepares, and organizes the appropriate equipment.
_____ 6. Applies tourniquet.
_____ 7. Selects site for venipuncture.
_____ 8. Loosens tourniquet.
_____ 9. Appropriately cleanses site with alcohol/acetone scrub.
_____ 10. Appropriately cleanses site using iodine ampule.
_____ 11. Appropriately cleanses collection container top with iodine.
_____ 12. Allows site to air dry.
_____ 13. Allows top of collection container to air dry.
_____ 14. Reapplies the tourniquet without contaminating the venipuncture site.
_____ 15. Appropriately completes venipuncture.
_____ 16. Appropriately discards needle in a needle disposal unit.
_____ 17. Appropriately discards biohazardous waste materials in biohazard receptacles.
_____ 18. Appropriately discards remaining waste materials.
_____ 19. Appropriately labels evacuated tube containing SPS.

Checklist:

Venipuncture of Artificial Arms for Blood Culture Specimen Collection #2

(A) Performed **(B) Needs Improvement** **(C) Not Performed**

Comments:

_____ 1. Washes hands. Dons gloves and gown.
_____ 2. Role play: Approaches patient.
_____ 3. Role play: Identifies patient.
_____ 4. Role play: Explains procedure to the patient.
_____ 5. Selects, prepares, and organizes the appropriate equipment.
_____ 6. Applies tourniquet.
_____ 7. Selects site for venipuncture.
_____ 8. Loosens tourniquet.
_____ 9. Appropriately cleanses site with alcohol/acetone scrub.
_____ 10. Appropriately cleanses site using iodine ampule.
_____ 11. Appropriately cleanses collection container top with iodine.
_____ 12. Allows site to air dry.
_____ 13. Allows top of collection container to air dry.
_____ 14. Reapplies the tourniquet without contaminating the venipuncture site.
_____ 15. Appropriately completes venipuncture.
_____ 16. Appropriately discards needle in a needle disposal unit.
_____ 17. Appropriately discards biohazardous waste materials in biohazard receptacles.
_____ 18. Appropriately discards remaining waste materials.
_____ 19. Appropriately labels evacuated tube containing SPS.

Checklist:

Venipuncture on Practice Patient for Blood Culture Specimen Collection

(A) Performed **(B) Needs Improvement** **(C) Not Performed**

Comments:

_____ 1. Washes hands. Dons gloves and gown.
_____ 2. Role play: Approaches patient.
_____ 3. Role play: Identifies patient.
_____ 4. Role play: Explains procedure to the patient.
_____ 5. Selects, prepares, and organizes equipment.
_____ 6. Applies tourniquet.
_____ 7. Selects site for venipuncture.
_____ 8. Loosens tourniquet.
_____ 9. Appropriately cleanses site with alcohol/acetone scrub.
_____ 10. Appropriately cleanses site using iodine ampule.
_____ 11. Appropriately cleanses top of collection container with iodine.
_____ 12. Allows site to air dry.
_____ 13. Allows top of container to air dry.
_____ 14. Reapplies the tourniquet without contaminating the venipuncture site.
_____ 15. Positions the holder between the thumb and index finger.
_____ 16. Uncaps the needle. Inspects the needle for manufacturer's defects.
_____ 17. Anchors the vein selected.
_____ 18. Inserts needle, bevel up, at correct angle.
_____ 19. Inserts needle in the same direction as the vein.
_____ 20. Pushes the evacuated tube onto the back of the needle without moving the needle.
_____ 21. Draws evacuated tubes in the appropriate order, if applicable.

Comments: **(A) Performed** **(B) Needs Improvement** **(C) Not Performed**

_____ 22. Removes the last evacuated tube from the back of the needle.
_____ 23. Places gauze over the puncture site.
_____ 24. Withdraws the needle. Instructs patient to apply pressure to the puncture site using sterile gauze.
_____ 25. Gently inverts the tubes with additives 5 to 10 times.
_____ 26. Labels tubes appropriately.
_____ 27. Labels tubes immediately following the draw.
_____ 28. Discards needle in needle disposal unit.
_____ 29. Discards materials contaminated with blood in biohazard bag.
_____ 30. Removes equipment and appropriately discards other waste materials.
_____ 31. Inspects puncture site; applies bandage, if necessary.
_____ 32. Removes gloves. Washes hands.
_____ 33. Leaves patient courteously.

Study Questions
Lab 17

1. Define bacteremia and septicemia. What is the difference between the 2 terms?

2. List and describe 3 containers used to collect and transport blood culture specimens.

3. What advantage(s) does each collection container in question #2 offer?

4. Define false positive and false negative. What collection errors may cause a false-positive blood culture result? What collection errors may cause a false-negative blood culture result?

5. In what order should the following tests be drawn: CBC, cardiac enzymes, blood culture, PT, and APTT?

6. How does blood culture specimen collection vary from that of a routine venipuncture?

LAB 18

Glucometer® Testing

Objective

To introduce bedside glucose testing procedures, using the Glucometer III® system

Equipment

Gloves; Gown; 70% isopropyl alcohol prep pads; Sterile gauze; Lancet; Glucometer III®; Glucofilm® test strips; Normal control solution; Abnormal control solution; Facial tissues; Needle disposal unit; Biohazard bag

Discussion

Many facilities are incorporating glucose testing at the patient's bedside. Bedside testing for glucose results in a markedly decreased turnaround time. The patient's glucose levels are available almost immediately after the blood specimen is collected. Additionally, the patient is subjected to a skin puncture rather than a venipuncture procedure. This may result in reduced patient discomfort and anxiety, particularly if the patient is difficult to draw by venipuncture. Finally, the volume of blood required for the analysis is much less for bedside testing than for routine testing using a venous sample.

The Glucometer® system is a reflectometer. The amount of glucose in a patient's blood specimen is directly proportional to the amount of light reflected off the test pad. The Glucometer® measures the amount of light reflected, calculates the amount of glucose present, and displays the patient's glucose level on the digital screen.

Quality Control

Strict adherence to established quality control procedures is critical to the success of any bedside glucose testing program. To ensure a quality program, phlebotomists (and any other health care worker performing bedside glucose testing) must follow the quality control guidelines established by the facility's supervisory personnel. If the patient's blood specimen is to be obtained by skin puncture, the phlebotomist must adhere to the standard quality control guidelines established for skin puncture procedures. Please refer to Lab #15 for a list of quality control guidelines for skin puncture procedures. In addition, glucose analysis often requires that the patient be fasting for quality results.

The patient must be interviewed prior to specimen collection to be sure that he or she properly prepared (in this case, fasted) before specimen collection.

Adherence to quality control procedures for maintaining the Glucometer® is also crucial to the success of a bedside glucose program. The instrument should be calibrated at least monthly. Calibration should be documented on a quality control chart.

In addition, normal and abnormal control solution must be analyzed each day patient testing is performed to ensure appropriate functioning of the glucose analyzer. Furthermore, every time a new lot number of reagent sticks is incorporated into use, the control tests must be repeated. The control test result must fall within a range specified by supervisory personnel. If a control value is outside the acceptable range, investigation into the procedure is required. Control values are plotted on a daily chart and reviewed by supervisory personnel. The supervisory personnel will interpret the control values for unacceptable results and patterns.

Procedure:
Glucometer® Testing

Checking the Instrument

1. Turn the instrument on by pressing the blue button.
2. Slide open the test well.
3. The display will read 60. Press the blue button. The display will begin to count down.
4. When the display reads 20, a beep will sound.
5. Insert the check paddle into the well with the checkmark on the handle positioned facing toward the digital display.
6. A result will appear on the digital display.
7. Compare the result on the display with the acceptable ranges printed on the insert included with the check paddle.
8. If the check paddle result is within the established range, the instrument is functioning properly.
10. Note the program number on the Glucofilm® bottle label.
11. Press the blue button until the number on the display matches the program number on the bottle label.

Running a Control Test

(Running a control test helps to ensure the accuracy of the test results.)

12. Remove a fresh Glucofilm® test strip from the bottle. Recap the bottle.
13. Remove the cap from the normal control solution.

14. Fold a facial tissue in quarters and place on a firm surface.
15. Place the Glucofilm® test strip with the reaction pad facing up on the facial tissue.
16. Slide open the test well.
17. The display will read 60. Apply a large drop of normal control to the pad on the test strip.
18. When the display reads 25, prepare the blot strip. At 20 seconds a beep will sound. Quickly blot the test pad with the folded facial tissue.
19. Immediately after blotting the test pad, insert the reagent strip into the test well. Slide the test well closed.
20. The control test result will appear on the display screen.
21. Compare the result on the display screen with the acceptable ranges for normal control. The acceptable ranges are printed on the package insert of the normal control. Record the control result on your result sheet.
22. Remove the test strip from the door and discard in a biohazard container.
23. Repeat steps 12 through 22, using the abnormal control solution.

Running a Patient Test

24. Following standard procedures, perform a skin puncture on your lab partner (refer to Lab #11, if necessary).
25. Wipe away the first drop of blood.
26. Squeeze the patient's finger to form a large drop of blood on the fingertip.
27. Follow steps 12 through 22, using patient blood obtained from your lab partner instead of control solution.
28. Record your results.
29. Discard the lancet in the needle disposal unit.
30. Discard the test strip and any other materials contaminated with blood in a biohazard container.
31. Press the on/off button to turn off the Glucometer III®.

Checklist:

Glucometer® Testing

(A) Performed **(B) Needs Improvement** **(C) Not Performed**

Comments:

_____ 1. Appropriately programs the Glucometer III®.
_____ 2. Prepares equipment prior to performing control test: removes reagent strip, folds facial tissue, opens normal control solution, positions reagent strip on facial tissue, opens test well.
_____ 3. Appropriately applies normal control solution to the reagent pad.
_____ 4. Presses start button on the Glucometer III®.
_____ 5. Appropriately blots excess normal control solution.
_____ 6. Appropriately places test strip in Glucometer III® for analysis.
_____ 7. Appropriately interprets results generated by Glucometer III®.
_____ 8. Repeats steps 2 through 7 using the abnormal control solution.
_____ 9. Washes hands. Dons gloves and gown.
_____ 10. Role play: Approaches patient.
_____ 11. Role play: Identifies patient.
_____ 12. Role play: Explains procedure. Interviews patient concerning preparation prior to specimen collection.
_____ 13. Selects, prepares, and organizes equipment.
_____ 14. Selects area for puncture site.
_____ 15. Gently massages finger chosen from hand to fingertip 3 to 4 times.
_____ 16. Appropriately applies heel warmer, if necessary.
_____ 17. Removes alcohol prep pad from package.
_____ 18. Cleanses the site in a circular motion beginning at the puncture site and moving outward.
_____ 19. Allows the site to air dry.
_____ 20. Holds the patient's finger securely.

Comments: **(A) Performed** **(B) Needs Improvement** **(C) Not Performed**

_____ 21. Appropriately positions the lancet.
_____ 22. Performs skin puncture.
_____ 23. Squeezes the finger to form first drop of blood.
_____ 24. Wipes away the first drop of blood.
_____ 25. Appropriately saturates test pad of the reagent strip with patient's blood.
_____ 26. Presses start button on the Glucometer III®.
_____ 27. Appropriately blots reagent strip with facial tissue.
_____ 28. Appropriately places reagent strip in Glucometer III®.
_____ 29. Provides appropriate postpuncture care to the patient.
_____ 30. Records patient results on result sheet.
_____ 31. Discards lancet in needle disposal unit.
_____ 32. Discards materials contaminated with blood in biohazard bag.
_____ 33. Appropriately discards other waste materials.
_____ 34. Inspects puncture site; applies bandage, if necessary.
_____ 35. Removes equipment.
_____ 36. Removes gloves and gown. Washes hands.
_____ 37. Leaves patient courteously.

Result Sheet:

Glucometer® Testing

Normal Control Lot #:________________

Expiration Date: ____________________

Result: ____

Is this result in an acceptable range? Why or why not? ____________________

____

Abnormal Control Lot #:_______________

Expiration Date: ____________________

Result: ____

Is this result in an acceptable range? Why or why not?____________________

____

Given the results of the control tests, what is the next appropriate step? ______

____

Patient Name: ____

Result: ____

Is this a normal or an abnormal result? __________________________________

____

Study Questions
Lab 18

1. Draw the chemical reaction that occurs on the test pad that is inserted into the Glucometer® for measurement.

2. What is the relationship between JCAHO, CAP, and quality control? ______

______

______

3. What advantage(s) is provided with a bedside glucose testing program over the customary laboratory analysis of glucose specimens? ______

______

4. What disadvantage(s) exists with a bedside glucose testing program? ______

______

5. Describe a hemalet. Explain what additional precautions must be taken when using a hemalet to ensure lancet sterility. ______

______

6. Outline the quality control program established at your facility for analyzing glucose on patient specimens using the Glucometer®. ______

______

______

LAB 19

Glucose Tolerance Testing

Objective

To gain expertise in performing skin punctures; to introduce the student to the process of administering a 3-hour glucose tolerance test; to gain expertise in operating the Glucometer®

Equipment

Gloves; Gown; 1 standard adult dose of glucose solution; Glucometer III®; 5 70% isopropyl alcohol prep pads; 5 sterile gauze pads; 5 safety flow lancets; 5 Glucofilm® test strips; 1 bottle of normal control solution; 1 bottle of abnormal control solution; Tissue paper (to blot reagent strips); 5 urine collection containers; Needle disposal unit; Biohazard bag

Discussion

Tolerance testing is performed when a patient exhibits symptoms suggesting abnormal metabolism of a particular analyte. In tolerance testing, the patient is given a measured amount of the substance suspected of causing the patient's symptoms, and the body's response is then measured. Glucose tolerance testing (GTT) is performed when a patient exhibits symptoms consistent with abnormal glucose metabolism. Conditions associated with abnormal glucose metabolism include diabetes mellitus and hypoglycemia.

Patient Preparation

Prior to a GTT, the patient should: eat regular, balanced meals for 3 days before the scheduled GTT; not eat, smoke, drink coffee or alcohol, or exercise strenuously for 12 hours before the beginning of the test; be advised that these activities will also be restricted throughout the test procedure; and be informed of the test procedure, reinforcing the length of time a patient must be at the testing site to complete the test.

Before initiating the GTT, fasting blood and urine specimens are obtained from the patient. Many facilities require that the fasting specimens be analyzed before beginning the GTT. If the glucose levels are beyond acceptable ranges for fasting specimens (too high or too low), the patient's physician is notified. Based on the results of the fasting specimen, the patient's physician decides whether or not to continue the test. For the purpose of the student lab, acceptable ranges of glucose levels for fasting blood specimens will be 2.8 to 8.9 mmol/L (50 to 160 mg/dL). Acceptable ranges of glucose levels for fasting urine levels are trace amounts or less.

Glucose Levels/Urine Specimens

For the purpose of this exercise, patient urine specimens will be analyzed using the glucose reagent strips and the color chart on the reagent bottle. The reaction pad on the reagent test strip is submerged in the patient's urine specimen. After 30 seconds, the reagent pads are blotted using facial tissue. The reaction is allowed to proceed (timed) for an additional 90 seconds. After the additional 90 seconds, the color of the reagent strip is matched against the color chart on the side of the reagent strip bottle. The level of glucose in the patient's urine is determined by matching the color of the reagent test pad to the appropriate color on the side of the reagent strip bottle.

Labeling

When labeling specimens obtained during a GTT, routine labeling practices should be practiced. In addition, the specimens, both urine and blood, should be labeled with the timing of the sample (eg, 1 hour, 2 hour, etc).

Urine specimens should have labels affixed to the specimen container (not the lid). Labels of urine specimens should contain all routine labeling information as well as the timing of the sample. If a patient is unable to void at a particular interval, the empty urine container should be labeled with all the appropriate information. "Patient unable to void" should be noted on the request form. In the student lab, the notation should be made on the result sheet.

Quality Control

To ensure quality test results in the glucose tolerance test procedure, the following quality control guidelines should be practiced.

1. All quality control guidelines for the collection of blood specimens by routine venipuncture or routine skin puncture (depending on which collection technique is used) should be followed.
2. The quality of test results is affected by the quality of patient preparation. The phlebotomist should be sure that the patient understands all of the instructions given before scheduling the test. The patient should be interviewed by the phlebotomist before the start of the test to ensure patient adherence to preparatory guidelines.
3. The patient should be encouraged to drink water throughout the procedure to ensure the availability of a urine specimen at each testing interval.

4. Blood specimens should be collected in a uniform manner (ie, either entirely by skin puncture or entirely by venipuncture). It is inappropriate, for example, for the blood specimen to be collected at the 30-minute interval by venipuncture and the specimen at the 60-minute interval by skin puncture. Clinically important differences are noted in the concentration of glucose when venous samples and skin puncture samples are analyzed and compared. Glucose levels are higher in skin puncture specimens than in venipuncture specimens. Consequently, switching collection techniques may cause a significant difference in glucose concentration, which is independent of the patient's ability to metabolize glucose.
5. Specimens should be collected as closely as possible to the assigned times. If a phlebotomist is not able to obtain a specimen at one of the specified intervals, the supervisor should be notified immediately.

Safety Considerations

Consult your instructor and/or supervisor for instruction on the glucose solution to be administered. Your instructor or supervisor may wish to substitute a placebo for the glucose solution.

If patients feel faint or nauseous, have them lie down and provide them with an emesis basin and towel. If the patient vomits, note the time and notify the patient's physician. If the patient vomits within the first 30 minutes of the procedure, the test is usually rescheduled. If the patient vomits 75 minutes into the test, the test is usually completed.

Follow all of the standard safety practices described in this workbook. If the protective gown becomes soiled with blood or body fluids at some point during the procedure, it should be discarded and replaced with a clean gown.

Assignment

Perform a 3-hour glucose tolerance test on your laboratory partner, using a glucose solution approved by your instructor and/or supervisor. Blood specimens are to be obtained by skin puncture and analyzed using the Glucometer III®. Record your results on the result sheet provided. Plot the glucose levels of your patient on the chart provided.

Procedure:

Glucose Tolerance Testing

1. Perform quality control check on Glucometer III®, using normal and abnormal control solution (refer to Lab #18).
2. Role play: Approach and identify patient following standard procedures.
3. Role play: Explain the GTT procedure to the patient. Be sure to include the following information in your explanation: the activities that were restricted as preparation for the test will continue to be restricted for the duration of the test; the test involves collecting a fasting blood and urine specimen, followed by the administration of a glucose solution; following administration of the glucose solution, several additional blood and urine specimens will be collected (a 3-hour test will require the collection of 4 specimens in addition to the fasting specimen); and the length of time required to complete the GTT for a 3-hour test is 3.5 to 4 hours.
4. Role play: Interview the patient to verify appropriate preparation. Be sure to inquire if the patient ate regular, balanced meals for 3 days prior to the scheduled GTT and did not eat, smoke, drink coffee or alcohol, or exercise strenuously for 12 hours before the beginning of the test.
5. Provide the patient with a urine collection container. Ask the patient to void in the container.
6. Label patient's urine specimen.
7. Perform a skin puncture on the patient. Wipe away the first drop of blood.
8. Place an appropriate amount of patient blood on Glucofilm® reagent strip.
9. Using the Glucometer III®, analyze the patient's blood sample for the level of glucose present (refer to Lab #18).

10. Record the result on the result sheet.
11. Analyze the patient's urine for glucose using a Glucofilm® reagent strip.
12. Record the results in the appropriate area of the result sheet. The level of glucose in the patient's urine should be reflected on the result sheet as negative, 1+, 2+, etc.
13. If the patient's glucose levels (on the fasting blood and urine specimens) are within acceptable ranges, proceed with the GTT.
14. Administer standard adult dose of glucose solution. Observe time. The patient must drink the entire dose within 5 minutes. Remain with the patient until he/she has completed drinking the solution. Observe time to: 1) ensure the patient has ingested the glucose solution within 5 minutes, and 2) begin timing the specimen collections from the time the patient has completely ingested the glucose solution. Remain with the patient until the entire glucose solution has been consumed.
15. Repeat steps 3 through 12 above at .5 hour following glucose administration, 1 hour following glucose administration, 2 hours following glucose administration, and 3 hours following glucose administration.
16. Record results on the result sheet.

Checklist:

Glucose Tolerance Testing

Comments:

(A) Performed **(B) Needs Improvement** **(C) Not Performed**

_____ 1. Washes hands. Dons gloves and gown.
_____ 2. Appropriately performs the check paddle test. Correctly interprets results.
_____ 3. Prepares equipment prior to performing control test (refer to Lab #18).
_____ 4. Appropriately applies normal control solution to the reagent pad.
_____ 5. Presses start button on the Glucometer III®.
_____ 6. Appropriately blots excess control solution.
_____ 7. Appropriately places test strip in the Glucometer III® for analysis.
_____ 8. Appropriately interprets the results generated by the Glucometer III®.
_____ 9. Repeats steps 3 to 8 using abnormal control solution.
_____ 10. Removes gloves. Washes hands. Dons a fresh pair of gloves.
_____ 11. Role play: Approaches patient.
_____ 12. Role play: Identifies patient.
_____ 13. Role play: Explains procedure.
_____ 14. Role play: Interviews patient to determine proper preparation for the glucose tolerance test.
_____ 15. Selects, prepares, and organizes skin puncture equipment.
_____ 16. Selects area for puncture site.
_____ 17. Gently massages finger chosen from hand to fingertip 3 to 4 times.
_____ 18. Appropriately applies heel warmer, if necessary.
_____ 19. Removes alcohol prep pad from the package.
_____ 20. Cleanses the site in a circular motion, beginning at the puncture site and moving outward.
_____ 21. Allows the site to air dry.
_____ 22. Holds the patient's finger securely.

Comments: **(A) Performed** **(B) Needs Improvement** **(C) Not Performed**

_____ 23. Appropriately positions the lancet.
_____ 24. Performs the skin puncture.
_____ 25. Squeezes the finger to form the first drop of blood.
_____ 26. Wipes away the first drop of blood, using a piece of sterile gauze.
_____ 27. Appropriately saturates the test pad of the reagent strip with the patient's blood (refer to Lab #18).
_____ 28. Presses the start button on the Glucometer III®.
_____ 29. Appropriately blots reagent strip with facial tissue (refer to Lab #18).
_____ 30. Appropriately places reagent strip in the reaction well of the Glucometer III®.
_____ 31. Discards the lancet in the needle disposal unit.
_____ 32. Discards materials contaminated with blood in the biohazard bag.
_____ 33. Appropriately discards other waste materials.
_____ 34. Inspects puncture site; applies bandage, if necessary.
_____ 35. Removes equipment.
_____ 36. Removes gloves. Washes hands.
_____ 37. Records patient results on the result sheet.
_____ 38. Provides the patient with a urine collection container.
_____ 39. Directs the patient to the restroom and asks the patient to void a urine specimen into the cup provided. Ensures the patient's privacy and leaves the restroom.
_____ 40. Washes hands. Dons gloves.
_____ 41. Appropriately labels the urine specimen provided.
_____ 42. Analyzes the patient's urine for glucose.
_____ 43. Appropriately records the result of the glucose analysis.
_____ 44. Interprets the results to determine whether or not to proceed with the glucose tolerance test.

Comments: **(A) Performed** **(B) Needs Improvement** **(C) Not Performed**

______ 45. Removes gloves. Washes hands.
______ 46. Administers glucose solution to the patient, if appropriate.
______ 47. Observes patient drinking the entire glucose solution.
______ 48. Times the ingestion of the glucose solution to ensure its completion within 5 minutes.
______ 49. Notes the time the glucose solution was completely imbibed by the patient.
______ 50. Washes hands. Dons gloves.
______ 51. Repeats steps 15 through 43, 30 minutes after the glucose solution was administered.
______ 52. Repeats steps 15 through 43, 60 minutes after the glucose solution was administered.
______ 53. Repeats steps 15 through 43, 120 minutes after the glucose solution was administered.
______ 54. Repeats steps 15 through 43, 180 minutes after the glucose solution was administered.
______ 55. Charts the results on the graph provided.

Result Sheet:

Glucose Tolerance Testing

Normal Control Lot #:________________

Expiration Date: ____________________

Result: ____

Abnormal Control Lot #:______________

Expiration Date: ____________________

Result: ____

Are the results of the normal and abnormal control acceptable? Why or why not?

____

Patient's Name: ____

Fasting Specimen Results: _____________________________________

Blood: ____

Urine: ____

Based on the results listed above, which of the following is the most appropriate course of action? (Check one)

________ Continue with the GTT

________ Contact the patient's physician before continuing with the GTT

Time glucose solution administered:_______________________________

Time administration of glucose completed: __________________________

Did the patient complete ingestion of glucose within 5 minutes? ____________

Complete the chart:

Timing of Sample	Time of Sample	Results/Blood	Results/Urine
.5 hr			
1 hr			
2 hr			
3 hr			

Graph the results.

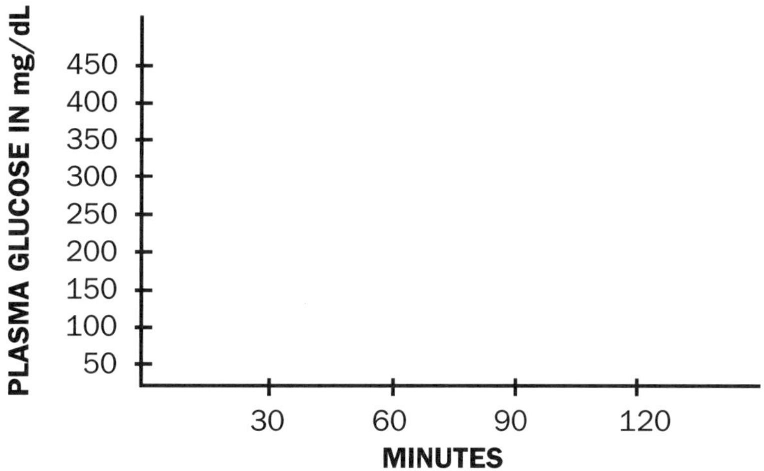

Study Questions
Lab 19

1. How does a GTT differ from a 2-hour postprandial? ________________________

____

2. When is a 1-hour postprandial most commonly ordered? ________________________

____

3. List and define at least 3 other types of tolerance tests. ________________________

____

____

____

4. How does each tolerance test listed in question #3 differ from a GTT?

____

____

5. Describe the sweat chloride test. Why would a sweat chloride test be ordered?

____

____

6. How is the dose of glucose solution determined? ________________________

____

____

LAB 20

Special Collection and Transport Techniques

Objective

To gain expertise in performing venipuncture; to introduce the collection of blood specimens for the cold agglutinin titer and the type and crossmatch; to introduce the special techniques of transport on ice and transport shielded from light

Equipment

Gloves; Gown; 4 needles; Holder; 2 10-mL red-top evacuated tubes; 1 blue-top evacuated tube; 1 SST evacuated tube; Tourniquet; 4 70% isopropyl alcohol prep pads; Sterile gauze; 37°C incubator; Crossmatch identification bracelet; Ice; Emesis basin or paper cup; Aluminum foil; Needle disposal unit; Biohazard bag

Cold Agglutinin

Cold agglutinin titers are ordered primarily by physicians to aid in making a differential diagnosis of primary atypical pneumonia. Low titers (1:16 or less) of cold agglutinins will be found in normal sera. The cold agglutinin response is related directly to the length and severity of a patient's illness. To prevent the stimulation of cold-reacting antibodies (agglutinins) outside of the test procedure, the collection vessel and sample must be maintained at 37°C.

Type and Crossmatch

Type and crossmatch tests are ordered prior to the transfusion of certain blood products. The standard procedure for type and crossmatch includes the following tests on a patient's blood specimen: ABO and Rh typing, antibody screen, and compatibility testing.

If blood transfusion is a possibility, the physician may elect to order a type and screen. Type and screen procedures include an ABO and Rh type and antibody screen only. The patient's blood sample is maintained in the blood bank for use if a crossmatch becomes necessary, as determined by the patient's physician.

Normal values for type and crossmatch procedures vary. Persons belong to one of the following groups: A, B, AB, or O. Persons are Rh positive or Rh negative. Antibody screens are usually negative. If the antibody screen is positive, the irregular antibody must be identified before blood can be issued for transfusion.

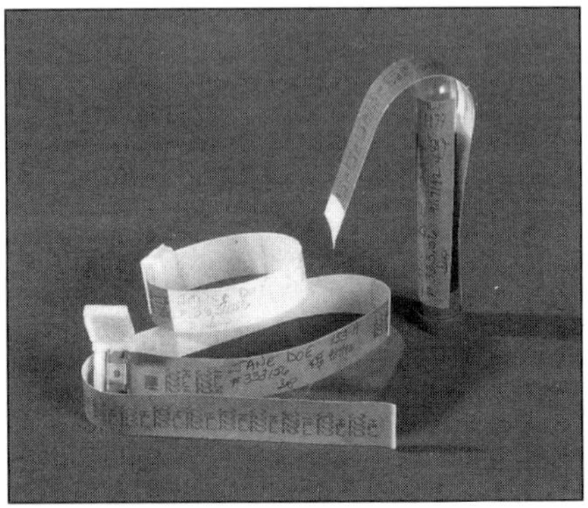

Figure 20-1 Crossmatch identification bracelet and corresponding label affixed to evacuated tube.

Although not mandated by regulatory agencies, some facilities incorporate the use of the crossmatch identification bracelet before collection of specimens for any type and crossmatch and type and screen procedures (**Fig. 20-1**). The crossmatch identification bracelet is available in a variety of colors. Prior to the collection of a blood specimen for type and crossmatch, patient identification information (patient's name, room number, hospital identification number, date and time of collection, and the phlebotomist's initials) is copied from the patient's hospital identification bracelet using a ballpoint pen. The crossmatch identification bracelet is affixed around the patient's wrist and secured using the plastic clamp. The crossmatch identification bracelet should be loose enough to

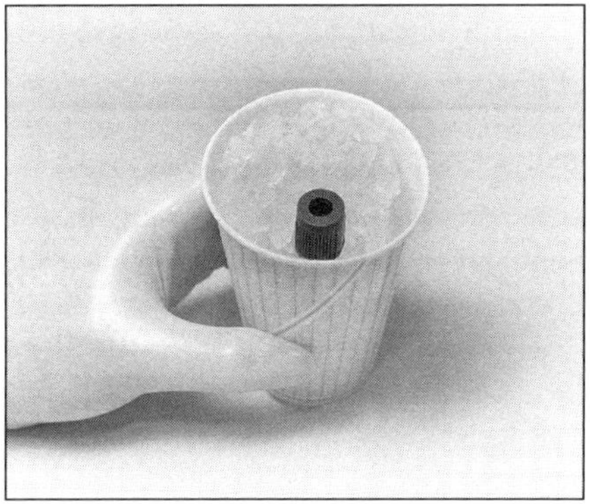

Figure 20-2 Transport of a chilled specimen on ice.

move freely but not too loose so that it may slip off the patient's wrist. A red- or pink-top evacuated tube is collected by routine venipuncture procedures.

After completing the venipuncture, the label is peeled off the crossmatch identification bracelet and affixed to the specimen tube. The identification numbers are detached from the bracelet and affixed to the side of the evacuated tube opposite the label. An identification number is peeled from the specimen tube and affixed to the requisition form. The identification numbers will be placed on each unit of blood (or blood products) tested and found appropriate for transfusion for that patient. The identification numbers will also appear on the transfusion report form to be completed at the time of transfusion. Before the transfusion is initiated, the patient's name, hospital number, and crossmatch identification numbers will be verified by the nurse.

The purpose of the crossmatch identification bracelet is to ensure proper patient identification, which is always necessary and crucial to the quality of specimen collected. When collecting blood specimens for any type and crossmatch or type and screen procedure, positive patient identification is imperative. Transfusion of a unit of blood or blood product that is an incorrect type can result in an adverse transfusion reaction, which can be fatal.

Chilled Specimens

Some tests require that the specimen be cooled immediately following collection to slow down metabolic processes that may alter some chemical values. Examples of tests requiring chilled specimens include acetone, ACTH, ammonia, catecholamines, fibrinogen, ketones, lactic acid, renin activity, and serum gastrin. To chill specimens immediately following collection, the specimen is transported on ice (**Fig. 20-2**).

Light-Sensitive Specimens

Certain values are altered if the blood specimen is exposed to light. Examples of light-sensitive entities in a blood sample include bilirubin, carotene, and erythrocyte protoporphyrin levels. Specimens drawn for these assays must be protected from the light. To accomplish this, the collection container must be shielded from the light by wrapping the specimen tube in aluminum foil (**Fig. 20-3**). Bilirubin samples may be obtained by skin puncture and collected in amber-colored capillary collection containers.

Procedure 1: Cold Agglutinin

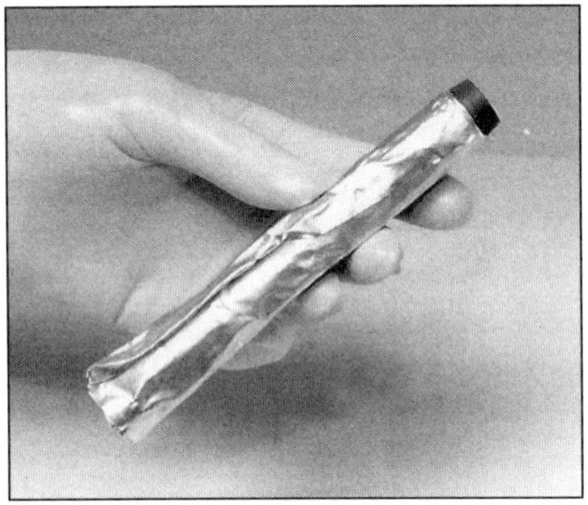

Figure 20-3 Transport of a light-sensitive specimen wrapped in foil.

1. Place a 10-mL red-top evacuated tube in a 37°C incubator for 30 minutes prior to venipuncture. This allows the collection tube to prewarm prior to collection of the blood specimen.
2. Transport the warmed tube in a 37°C portable incubator (or in your closed hand) to the patient's bedside.
3. Perform a routine venipuncture and collect a 10-mL red-top evacuated tube.
4. Transport the specimen to the appropriate department of the laboratory in the portable 37°C incubator or in the closed hand of the phlebotomist. (Most facilities perform cold agglutinin titers in the immunology department.)
5. Role play: Inform the technologist on duty that a specimen for cold agglutinin titer has been collected and placed in the 37°C incubator. If the technologist on duty is unaware that a specimen has arrived for cold agglutinin testing, the specimen will not be processed. If the specimen is not processed appropriately, it will be useless for testing and will have to be redrawn.
6. Log the specimen for cold agglutinin titer (#14) on the Venipuncture Record Sheet (Lab #16). Have your instructor initial the record sheet, indicating that the specimen for cold agglutinin titer was collected appropriately.

Quality Assurance

The phlebotomist should adhere to quality control guidelines for routine venipuncture. In addition, gel separation tubes are not acceptable for collection of specimens for cold agglutinin titers. Because the patient's red blood cells are used during the test procedure, collection of specimens in these tubes would contaminate the red blood cells, rendering them useless for testing. It is important that the collection tube and the collected specimen be maintained at 37°C. Allowing the specimen to cool will cause some cold agglutinins to react outside of the test procedure, which would introduce error into the procedure. Agglutination or hemolysis in the cold agglutinin titer is considered to be a positive result. Therefore, the phlebotomist should be careful not to hemolyze the specimen.

Procedure 2: Crossmatch

1. Assemble equipment for routine venipuncture, including a 10-mL red-top evacuated tube and a crossmatch identification bracelet.
2. Identify patient, using the 2-step method of patient identification.
3. Use a ballpoint pen to copy patient identification from the patient's hospital identification bracelet to the crossmatch identification bracelet. The following information should be included: patient's full name (first and last name); patient's hospital identification number; patient's room number; date of specimen collection; time of specimen collection; and phlebotomist's initials. Press hard enough with the pen so the information will carry through the carbon onto the bracelet.
4. Place the crossmatch identification bracelet on the patient's wrist and secure it by pinching the white clasp around the band. The band should be secure enough not to slide off, but loose enough to move freely around the patient's wrist.
5. Follow routine venipuncture procedures to collect a 10-mL red- or pink-top evacuated tube.
6. Specimens must always be labeled at the patient's bedside before leaving the patient. Peel the label off the crossmatch identification band and attach it to the specimen tube.
7. Detach the identification numbers from the crossmatch identification band by tearing the numbers off at the clasp. Remove the paper backing from the strip of identification numbers. Affix the strip of identification numbers to the specimen tube on the side of the tube opposite the label.

8. Record the specimen (#15) on the Venipuncture Record Sheet (Lab #16). Remove one of the identification numbers and place it on the log sheet. Have your instructor initial the record sheet, indicating that the specimen was appropriately collected.

Quality Control

The most important step in collecting a blood specimen for type and screen or type and crossmatch tests is correct patient identification. If a patient does not have a hospital identification wristband, request that one be prepared by the nursing staff. Insist that the hospital identification wristband be affixed to the patient's wrist before drawing the specimen. Hospital identification bracelets must be affixed to the patient's body to be acceptable forms of patient identification. Identification cards affixed over a patient's bed, identification bracelets affixed to a patient's bed, or verbal identification from another health care worker are unacceptable forms of patient identification.

When collecting specimens for type and screen or type and crossmatch procedures, be careful not to hemolyze the sample. When performing any type and screen or type and crossmatch procedures, a positive reaction is the presence of either agglutination of red blood cells or hemolysis. Consequently, it is inappropriate to begin testing with a hemolyzed specimen.

Gel separation tubes are not acceptable for the collection of specimens for any type and screen or type and crossmatch procedures. The patient's red blood cells are used during a type and screen or type and crossmatch procedure. The gel found in these tubes would coat the red blood cells, rendering them useless for testing. Blood specimens collected in evacuated tubes containing additives that bind calcium (lavender- or blue-top tubes) are inappropriate for use in type and crossmatch procedures.

Procedure 3: Chilled Specimens

1. The assignment is to collect a specimen for fibrinogen assay.
2. Select the appropriate equipment.
3. Prepare a cup of ice for transport of the blood specimen. Obtain ice from an appropriate source. (In the clinical setting, it is appropriate to ask at the nurse's station for ice. In the training setting, ask your instructor for ice.) Place the ice in a paper cup or an emesis basin. Bring the cup of ice (or emesis basin of ice) to the patient's bedside.
4. Collect the specimen, following routine venipuncture procedures.
5. Label the sample, following standard labeling procedures. Immediately after labeling the sample, submerge it in the ice.
6. Transport to the appropriate department.
7. Role play: Inform the technologist on duty that a specimen for fibrinogen assay has been delivered to the department.
8. Record the specimen (#16) on the Venipuncture Record Sheet (Lab #16). Have your instructor initial the record sheet, indicating that the specimen was appropriately collected and transported.

Procedure 4: Light-Sensitive Specimens

1. The assignment is to collect a specimen for carotene assay.
2. Select the appropriate equipment for a routine venipuncture.
3. Prepare for the special transport of the specimen by obtaining a piece of aluminum foil. The aluminum foil should be large enough to completely wrap the specimen tube.
4. Collect the blood specimen, following routine venipuncture procedures.
5. Label the specimen, following routine labeling procedures. Immediately after labeling the specimen, wrap it in aluminum foil.
6. Transport the wrapped specimen to the appropriate department for analysis.
7. Record the specimen (#17) on the Venipuncture Record Sheet (Lab #16). Have your instructor initial the record sheet, indicating that the specimen was appropriately collected and protected from the light.

Checklist: Special Collection and Transport Techniques

(A) Performed (B) Needs Improvement (C) Not Performed

Comments:

Cold Agglutinin

_____ 1. Selects appropriate tube for collection of specimen.
_____ 2. Appropriately warms tube.
_____ 3. Appropriately transports tube to patient's bedside.
_____ 4. Appropriately collects specimen by routine venipuncture.
_____ 5. Appropriately transports tube to laboratory.
_____ 6. Informs appropriate personnel that a cold agglutinin titer was placed in the 37°C incubator.

Type and Crossmatch

_____ 1. Prepares to perform a routine venipuncture.
_____ 2. Appropriately identifies patient.
_____ 3. Copies appropriate information onto crossmatch identification bracelet.
_____ 4. Appropriately places crossmatch identification bracelet on patient's wrist.
_____ 5. Follows routine venipuncture procedures to collect the specimen.
_____ 6. Collects specimen in an appropriate tube.
_____ 7. Removes label from the crossmatch identification bracelet and appropriately positions it on the specimen collected.
_____ 8. Detaches identification numbers from the crossmatch identification bracelet.
_____ 9. Affixes the identification numbers onto the specimen tube.

Transport of Chilled Specimens

_____ 1. Prepares to perform a routine venipuncture.
_____ 2. Selects the appropriate collection tube.
_____ 3. Prepares a cup of ice for transport of the specimen.
_____ 4. Collects blood specimen, following routine venipuncture procedures.

Comments: **(A) Performed** **(B) Needs Improvement** **(C) Not Performed**

_____ 5. Appropriately submerges specimen in ice for transport.
_____ 6. Delivers specimen to the appropriate department.
_____ 7. Informs appropriate personnel of the iced specimen.

Light-Sensitive Specimens

_____ 1. Prepares to perform a routine venipuncture.
_____ 2. Obtains a piece of aluminum foil, sufficient in size to accommodate the entire specimen tube.
_____ 3. Collects the blood specimen, following routine venipuncture procedures.
_____ 4. Wraps the labeled specimen tube in aluminum foil.

Study Questions
Lab 20

1. What do the results of a high cold agglutinin titer suggest? ______

______

2. What is *Mycoplasma pneumoniae*? ______

______

3. Accurate patient identification is absolutely necessary whenever a blood specimen is collected. What consequences may patients suffer if they are transfused with a unit of incompatible blood? ______

______

______

4. What is the most common cause of fatal hemolytic transfusion reactions?

______

5. Why is hemolysis unacceptable for both cold agglutinin and crossmatch samples?

______

______

6. How does cold agglutinin specimen collection vary from a routine venipuncture procedure? ______

______

7. How does type and crossmatch specimen collection differ from a routine venipuncture procedure? ______

______

LAB 21

Syringes

Objective

To introduce venipuncture incorporating the use of a syringe

Equipment

Tourniquet; Gloves; Gown; 70% isopropyl alcohol prep pad; Sterile gauze; 10-mL syringe; Thrombo Wellcotest tube; One 4-mL red-top evacuated tube; Needle disposal unit; Biohazard bag

Discussion

Some patients may be difficult to draw successfully using a routine evacuated tube system. Examples of such patient population groups include geriatric patients, pediatric patients, oncology patients, and burn victims. These patient groups may have tiny and/or fragile veins, which cannot withstand the vacuum pressure of standard-size (or pediatric-size) evacuated tubes. The syringe affords the phlebotomist more control over the amount of pressure exerted on a tiny and/or fragile vein during the venipuncture procedure. Evacuated tubes contain a vacuum strong enough to withdraw a specific volume of blood. As soon as the stopper is punctured, the entire strength of the vacuum is activated. The vacuum may be sufficient to cause a patient's vein to collapse. Syringes do not contain a vacuum but are filled by pulling back on the plunger, allowing blood to flow into the barrel of the syringe. The force exerted on the inside of the blood vessel may be increased or decreased by pulling the plunger faster or slower. Therefore, the amount of pressure exerted on the inside of the vein may be controlled by the phlebotomist to a certain extent. The phlebotomist may control the rate at which blood is withdrawn and thereby prevent a patient's veins from collapsing during blood specimen collection. This is advantageous when drawing blood from patients who have veins that are difficult to access. Many times, the ability to control the amount of pressure exerted on tiny and/or fragile veins will provide the phlebotomist with a successful procedure.

Quality Control

When collecting blood by syringe, the phlebotomist should follow the standard procedures for quality specimen collection by venipuncture. In addition, the following considerations must be made:

1. To avoid hemolyzing the specimen:
   a. Two methods are used for transferring blood from the collection syringe to the appropriate evacuated tube. Both are designed to prevent hemolysis of the blood specimen during transfer to evacuated tubes. Follow the procedure at your facility to aliquot specimen collected by syringe into the appropriate evacuated tube.

1) Remove the needle from the collection syringe, unstopper the evacuated tube, and depress the plunger of the syringe to aliquot the blood into the evacuated tube.
2) Insert the needle of the collection syringe through the stopper of the evacuated tube. Angle the needle toward the side of the tube and allow the vacuum to pull the blood into the tube. Do NOT depress the plunger. If this is the procedure followed at your facility, use a needle of sufficient size. Appropriate sizes are 21- or 22-gauge needles for transferring blood from the collection syringe to evacuated tubes.

b. The plunger should not be pulled back too forcefully, because this may cause the patient's veins to collapse or may hemolyze the specimen.

c. Be sure the needle is fitted securely onto the syringe. A loose-fitting needle may cause frothing of the specimen, resulting in a hemolyzed specimen.

2. If multiple evacuated tubes must be filled from one syringe, the order of draw is critical to quality test results. The appropriate order of draw is as follows: first, aseptic delivery of blood specimen into the blood culture bottle; second, sodium citrate tubes for coagulation studies; third, any other anticoagulated tube; and last, any tubes without anticoagulant additives.

Procedure: Syringes

1. Wash hands. Don gloves and gown.
2. Approach, identify, and interview the patient following standard procedures.
3. Select, prepare, and organize equipment. To prepare the syringe, remove it from the manufacturer's packaging. Move the plunger up and down in the barrel of the syringe several times (this will help to ensure ease of movement during the venipuncture). Push the plunger into the syringe prior to venipuncture. Be sure the plunger is completely depressed into the syringe barrel.
4. Secure the tourniquet.

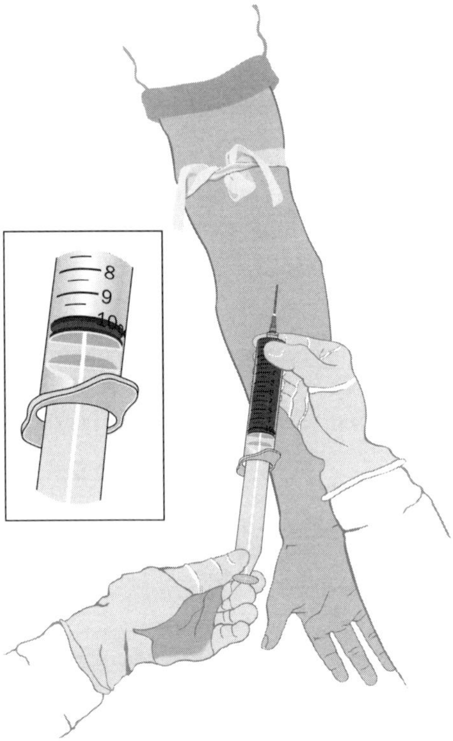

Figure 21-1 Pull the plunger back to collect the blood. Inset, 10-mL graduation on the syringe.

5. Select a venipuncture site by palpating for a vein.
6. Release the tourniquet.
7. Cleanse the site with the alcohol prep pad (refer to Lab #16).
8. Allow the site to air dry.
9. Reapply the tourniquet. Be sure that the ends of the tourniquet do not touch the cleansed venipuncture site.
10. Be sure the plunger of the syringe is completely pushed into the barrel of the syringe.
11. Uncap the needle. Inspect the needle for manufacturing defects.
12. Anchor the vein (refer to Lab #16).
13. Position the needle appropriately.
14. Insert the needle (bevel up). Often, if the needle is in the vein, a small amount of blood will appear in the hub of the needle.
15. While holding the needle absolutely still, pull back slowly but steadily on the plunger (refer to Lab #16).
16. Pull back on the plunger until 10 mL of blood has entered the syringe. Most syringes have a double ring on the plunger. When the ring closest to the needle rests on the 10-mL graduation, the syringe contains 10 mL of blood. If the plunger contains a double ring and a point, it should be pulled back until the point rests on the 10-mL graduation (**Fig. 21-1**).
17. Release the plunger. Untie the tourniquet.
18. Place a piece of gauze over the venipuncture site.
19. Withdraw the needle from the patient's arm.
20. Insert the needle through the stopper of the Thrombo Wellcotest tube. Allow the vacuum from the evacuated tube to pull the blood specimen into the tube. When the vacuum is exhausted, pull the needle from the tube.

21. Insert the needle through the stopper of the red-top tube. Allow the vacuum from the evacuated tube to pull the blood specimen into the tube. When the vacuum is exhausted, pull the needle from the red-top tube. Do not inject the blood from the syringe into either tube.

22. Dispose of the needle and syringe in an appropriate needle disposal unit.

23. Gently invert evacuated tubes containing additives 5 to 10 times.

24. Label the filled evacuated tubes following standard labeling procedures.

25. Record the specimen on the Venipuncture Record Sheet (Lab #16). Fill in the appropriate information. Allow the instructor to initial the record sheet.

Checklist: Syringe Draw

(A) Performed **(B) Needs Improvement** **(C) Not Performed**

Comments:

_____ 1. Washes hands. Dons gloves and gown.
_____ 2. Role play: Approaches patient.
_____ 3. Role play: Identifies patient using 2-step method.
_____ 4. Role play: Explains procedure. Interviews patient concerning preparation guidelines, if appropriate.
_____ 5. Selects, prepares, and organizes equipment.
_____ 6. Positions patient's arm.
_____ 7. Applies tourniquet.
_____ 8. Selects venipuncture site.
_____ 9. Loosens tourniquet.
_____ 10. Cleanses venipuncture site with alcohol. Allows site to air dry.
_____ 11. Reapplies tourniquet.
_____ 12. Anchors vein.
_____ 13. Smoothly inserts needle bevel up.
_____ 14. Slowly and steadily pulls back on the plunger of the syringe.

Comments: **(A) Performed** **(B) Needs Improvement** **(C) Not Performed**

_____14. Releases the tourniquet when an adequate amount of specimen has been collected.
_____16. Places gauze over the puncture site and smoothly withdraws the needle.
_____17. Directs the patient to apply pressure to the puncture site.
_____18. Inserts needle through the stopper of the Thrombo Wellcotest tube.
_____19. Appropriately withdraws the needle and inserts it through the stopper of the red-top evacuated tube.
_____20. Withdraws the needle from the red-top tube and disposes of the needle and syringe in an appropriate needle disposal unit.
_____21. Inverts the Thrombo Wellcotest tube gently at least 5 to 10 times.
_____22. Inspects puncture site; applies bandage, if necessary.
_____23. Labels the tubes appropriately.
_____24. Discards materials contaminated with blood in biohazard bag.
_____25. Removes equipment.
_____26. Removes gloves. Washes hands.
_____27. Leaves patient courteously.

Study Questions
Lab 21

1. What advantage can a syringe offer over an evacuated tube system when collecting blood specimens from patients with very small veins? ____________

____

2. List at least 3 types of patients who may require use of a syringe to obtain a blood specimen. ____________

____

3. List at least 3 ways a specimen drawn by syringe may become hemolyzed.

____

____

4. What is the rationale for the order of draw to be followed after collecting blood by syringe? ____________

____

5. Define disseminated intravascular coagulation (DIC). ____________

____

6. Would the following test results be increased or decreased if a patient had DIC?

- Fibrinogen: ____________
- Platelet Count: ____________
- Fibrinogen Degradation Products: ____________
- Prothrombin Time: ____________
- Activated Partial Thromboplastin Time: ____________

LAB 22

Venipuncture With the Use of the Winged Infusion Needle

Objective

To introduce incorporating the winged infusion needle into the standard venipuncture procedure

Equipment

Gloves; Gown; 70% isopropyl alcohol prep pad; Sterile gauze pad; Tourniquet; Winged infusion needle/Syringe draw; Syringe; Winged infusion needle/Evacuated tube draw; One 4-mL red-top evacuated tube; One 4-mL lavender-top evacuated tube; Bandage; Tape; Artificial hand; Needle disposal unit; Biohazard bag

Discussion

Some phlebotomists prefer to collect blood specimens from patients with tiny, fragile veins through the use of a winged infusion needle instead of a syringe. Patient groups who may be easier to draw by the use of a winged infusion needle include pediatric patients, geriatric patients, oncology patients, and burn victims.

Winged infusion needles are preferable to standard venipuncture needles when drawing from tiny veins because they are commercially available in very small gauges (23 and 25 gauge). Small needles are easier to insert into tiny veins. In addition, winged infusion needles can adapt to both a syringe (**Fig. 22-1**) or a pediatric tube holder (**Fig. 22-2**). Both of these methods of collection are less likely to collapse a vein because the exertion of vacuum pressure is significantly lessened (as compared to the vacuum in a standard-size evacuated tube).

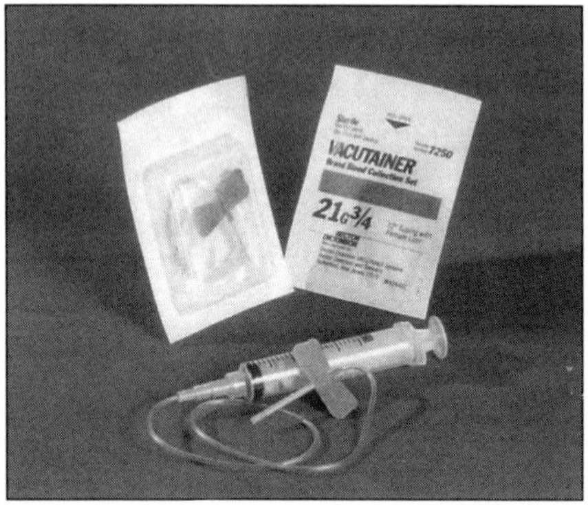

Figure 22-1 Winged infusion needle attached to a syringe.

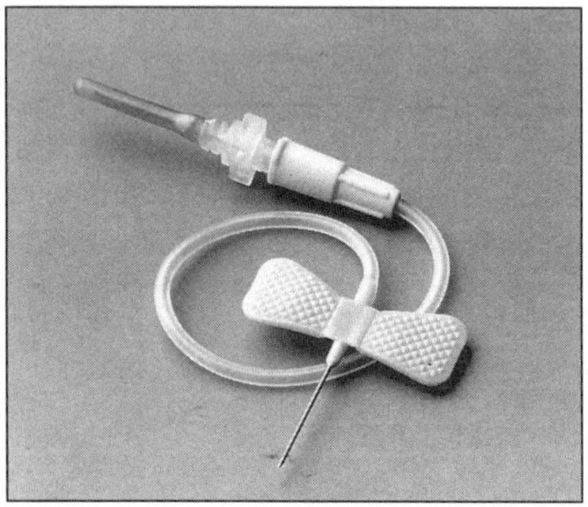

Figure 22-2 Winged infusion needle with evacuated tube attachment. (Photo courtesy of Becton Dickinson)

Alternative Venipuncture Sites

Sometimes, it is very difficult to locate a vein suitable for venipuncture in the antecubital fossa of a patient's arm. The appropriate course of action is to inspect the patient's other arm for a suitable vein. In the event that neither arm provides a vein suitable for venipuncture, the phlebotomist may then consider using a vein in the patient's hand or wrist.

Hand veins are more difficult to access than veins in the antecubital fossa because they are generally smaller. In addition, hand veins are not as well anchored by surrounding musculature as those in the antecubital fossa. Consequently, they have a tendency to move or "roll" when the needle is inserted. The phlebotomist should exercise extra care when anchoring a vein located in the hand or wrist to prevent it from moving during insertion of the needle (**Fig. 22-3**).

If a patient's hands and wrists are evaluated as potential venipuncture sites, and no suitable veins are found, some facilities will authorize phlebotomists to use veins located in the patient's ankles or feet. Always check the policy at your facility BEFORE performing venipuncture on a foot or ankle vein. The concerns related to venipuncture of veins in a patient's hands or wrists also have application for veins in the patient's ankles or feet. Both the hands and the feet have increased amounts of bacteria on their surface, as compared to the antecubital fossa. The phlebotomist should thoroughly cleanse the puncture site prior to venipuncture. If a vein in a patient's hand, wrist, foot, or ankle is chosen, a winged infusion needle or a syringe should be used because they often will accommodate smaller veins better than a standard evacuated tube assembly.

Quality Control

Follow standard quality control procedures outlined for routine venipuncture and collection of blood specimens by syringe (refer to Labs #16 and #21). Additionally, consult the procedure manual at your facility concerning the use of feet and ankle veins as potential sites for routine venipuncture.

Procedure 1: Venipuncture/Winged Infusion Needle/Syringe

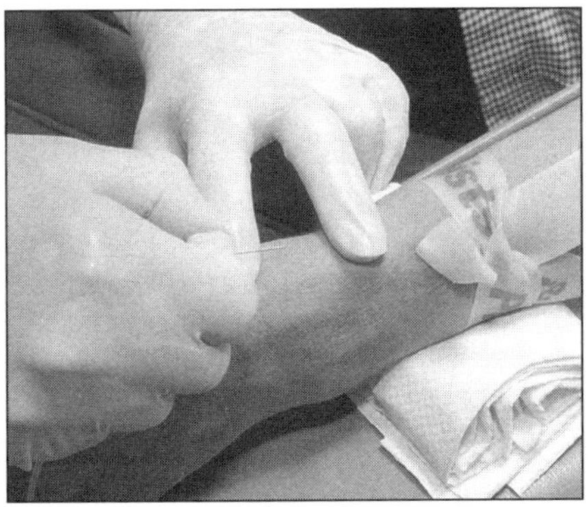

Figure 22-3 Proper anchoring of hand and wrist veins for venipuncture.

1. Select and organize equipment.
2. Approach and identify patient using standard procedures.
3. Select and prepare venipuncture site.
4. Prepare equipment. Remove the winged infusion needle from its packaging. Remove the syringe from its packaging. Move the plunger back and forth in the barrel of the syringe several times. Remove the needle from the syringe by twisting it off. SAVE THE SYRINGE NEEDLE! The syringe needle will be used to aliquot patient specimen from the syringe into evacuated tubes. Attach the syringe securely to the holder at the end of the tubing from the winged infusion needle.
5. Apply the tourniquet.
6. Select a venipuncture site by palpating for a vein.
7. Release the tourniquet.
8. Tear off 2 pieces of tape and attach one end of the tape on a surface where it is easily accessible.
9. Cleanse the site with the alcohol prep pad.
10. Allow the site to air dry.

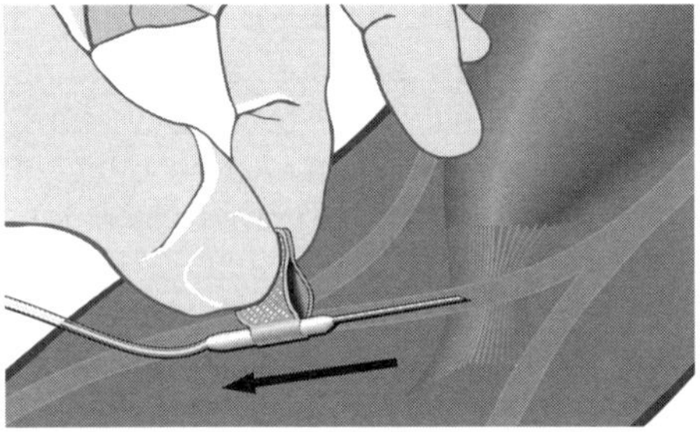

Figure 22-4 Bend wings of winged infusion needle together when withdrawing the needle.

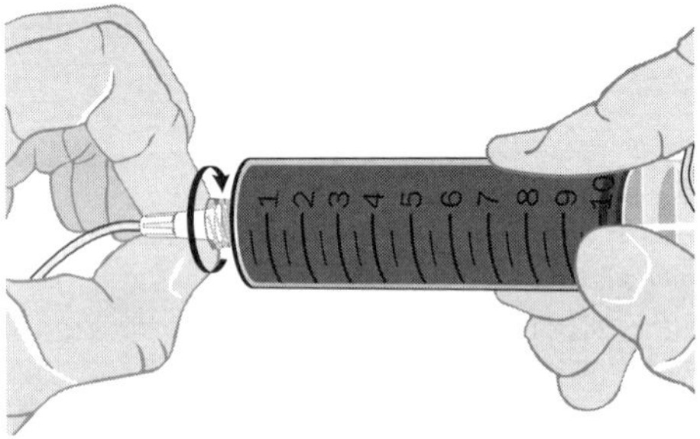

Figure 22-5 Unscrew the syringe from the tubing.

11. Reapply the tourniquet.
12. Be sure the plunger of the syringe is entirely depressed into the barrel.
13. Uncap the needle and inspect for manufacturing defects.
14. Anchor the vein.
15. Position the needle appropriately (refer to Lab #16).
16. Bend the wings together over the needle and insert it, bevel up.
17. Allow the wings of the needle to unbend and rest on the patient's arm. Place a piece of tape over the wings of the needle to secure it. The second piece of tape is a spare in the event of a misstep with the first piece.
18. Pull back on the plunger of the syringe until 8 mL has been collected.
19. Release the plunger. Untie the tourniquet.
20. Remove the tape from the wings of the needle.
21. Bend the wings of the needle together; withdraw the needle from the patient's arm (**Fig. 22-4**).
22. Remove the syringe from the tube by unscrewing the syringe until it is free of the tubing (**Fig. 22-5**).
23. Discard the winged infusion needle in an appropriate needle disposal unit.
24. Replace the needle originally packaged with the syringe onto the syringe.
25. Uncap the needle.
26. Insert the needle through the stopper of the lavender-top evacuated tube. Allow the vacuum to pull the blood into the evacuated tube. When the vacuum has been exhausted, withdraw the needle from the lavender-top evacuated tube. Repeat the procedure on the red-top evacuated tube.
27. Dispose of the needle and syringe in an appropriate needle disposal unit.
28. Gently invert the lavender-top tube 5 to 10 times.
29. Label the filled evacuated tubes following standard labeling procedures.

Procedure 2: Venipuncture/ Winged Infusion Needle/Evacuated Tube Holder

1. Select and organize equipment.
2. Approach and identify patient using standard procedures.
3. Prepare equipment. Open package containing winged infusion needle. Attach the evacuated tube holder onto the end of the tubing attached to the needle. Select one 4-mL red-top and one 4-mL lavender-top tube.
4. Apply the tourniquet around the patient's forearm, halfway between the wrists and the elbow.
5. Select a venipuncture site by palpating for a vein.
6. Release the tourniquet.
7. Tear off 2 pieces of tape and attach one end of the tape on a surface where it is easily accessible.
8. Cleanse the site with the alcohol prep pad.
9. Allow the site to air dry.
10. Reapply the tourniquet.
11. Grasp the needle by bending the wings together.
12. Uncap the needle and inspect for manufacturing defects.
13. Anchor the vein.
14. Position the needle appropriately (refer to Lab #16).
15. Insert the needle, bevel up.
16. Allow the wings of the needle to unbend and rest on the patient's arm. Place a piece of tape over the wings of the needle to secure it. The second piece is a spare in the event of a misstep with the first piece.
17. Push the red-top evacuated tube onto the needle secured by the holder. Allow it to fill.
18. Remove the red-top tube and replace it with the lavender-top tube. Allow the lavender-top tube to completely fill. Remove the tube from the needle.
19. Untie the tourniquet. Place gauze over the venipuncture site.
20. Remove the tape from the winged infusion needle.
21. Bend the wings together and withdraw the needle (see **Fig. 22-4**).

22. Dispose of the needle in an appropriate needle disposal unit.
23. Gently invert the lavender-top tube 5 to 10 times.
24. Label the tubes following standard labeling procedures.

Assignment

Perform each of these procedures on an artificial hand. Once the student feels confident in performing each procedure, the student may perform them for the instructor. The student's competency will be assessed by the instructor, using the checklists.

Checklist: Venipuncture/Winged Infusion Needle/Syringe

Comments:

(A) Performed **(B) Needs Improvement** **(C) Not Performed**

_____ 1. Washes hands. Dons gloves and gown.
_____ 2. Role play: Approaches patient.
_____ 3. Role play: Identifies patient.
_____ 4. Role play: Explains procedure. Interviews patient concerning preparation guidelines, if appropriate.
_____ 5. Selects, prepares, and organizes equipment.
_____ 6. Positions patient's arm.
_____ 7. Applies tourniquet.
_____ 8. Selects venipuncture site.
_____ 9. Loosens tourniquet.
_____ 10. Cleanses venipuncture site with alcohol.
_____ 11. Reapplies tourniquet.
_____ 12. Anchors vein.
_____ 13. Bends the wings of the winged infusion needle together and smoothly inserts the needle, bevel up.

Comments: **(A) Performed** **(B) Needs Improvement** **(C) Not Performed**

_____ 14. Secures the wings of the needle with tape.
_____ 15. Slowly and steadily pulls back on the plunger of the syringe.
_____ 16. When an adequate amount of specimen has been collected, releases the tourniquet.
_____ 17. Places gauze over the puncture site and smoothly withdraws the needle. Directs patient to apply pressure to the puncture site.
_____ 18. Removes syringe from winged infusion apparatus.
_____ 19. Reattaches syringe needle onto syringe.
_____ 20. Appropriately fills the lavender-top tube.
_____ 21. Appropriately fills the red-top tube.
_____ 22. Appropriately inverts lavender-top tube.
_____ 23. Appropriately labels specimens.
_____ 24. Checks puncture site to ascertain whether bleeding has stopped. Applies bandage, if needed.
_____ 25. Discards needles in needle disposal unit.
_____ 26. Discards materials contaminated with blood in biohazard bag.
_____ 27. Removes gloves. Washes hands.
_____ 28. Leaves patient courteously.

Checklist:

Venipuncture/ Winged Infusion Needle/Evacuated Tube Holder

Comments:

(A) Performed **(B) Needs Improvement** **(C) Not Performed**

_____ 1. Washes hands. Dons gloves and gown.
_____ 2. Role play: Approaches patient.
_____ 3. Role play: Identifies patient.
_____ 4. Role play: Explains procedure. Interviews patient concerning preparation guidelines, if appropriate.
_____ 5. Selects, prepares, and organizes equipment.
_____ 6. Positions patient's arm.
_____ 7. Applies tourniquet around patient's forearm.
_____ 8. Selects venipuncture site.
_____ 9. Loosens tourniquet.
_____ 10. Cleanses venipuncture site with alcohol.
_____ 11. Reapplies tourniquet.
_____ 12. Anchors vein.
_____ 13. Bends wings of the winged infusion needle together and smoothly inserts the needle, bevel up.
_____ 14. Pushes the red-top evacuated tube onto the needle in the holder.
_____ 15. Allows the tube to fill.
_____ 16. Pulls the filled tube off the needle in the holder.
_____ 17. Pushes the lavender-top tube onto the needle in the holder.
_____ 18. Releases tourniquet.
_____ 19. Places a gauze over the puncture site.
_____ 20. Removes the tape from the wings of the needle.
_____ 21. Bends the wings of the needle together.
_____ 22. Smoothly withdraws the needle.
_____ 23. Directs patient to apply pressure to the puncture site.
_____ 24. Discards the needle in the appropriate waste receptacle.

Comments: **(A) Performed** **(B) Needs Improvement** **(C) Not Performed**

_____ 25. Gently inverts the lavender-top tube 5 to 10 times.
_____ 26. Labels the tubes following standard labeling procedures.
_____ 27. Discards materials contaminated with blood in the biohazard bag.
_____ 28. Appropriately discards other waste materials.
_____ 29. Removes equipment. Applies bandage to puncture site, if necessary.
_____ 30. Removes gloves. Washes hands.
_____ 31. Leaves patient courteously.

Study Questions

Lab 22

1. Winged infusion needles may be attached to a syringe or a pediatric tube holder. Which collection method do you prefer? Explain.

2. How does pediatric blood collection by venipuncture differ from adult venipuncture?

3. List and describe at least 3 methods of blood collection site immobilization.

4. When using small needles to draw pediatric patients, what specimen quality concerns should the phlebotomist have?

5. What extra patient safety considerations must be made for pediatric patients?

LAB 23

Allen Test/Arterial Puncture Site Preparation/Collection of Capillary Blood Gases

Objective

To introduce the Allen Test procedure; to introduce the procedure for arterial puncture site preparation prior to the collection of blood gases; to introduce the specimen collection procedure for capillary blood gases

Equipment

Gloves; Gown; Heel warmer; Heparinized large-bore capillary tubes; Seals for the large-bore capillary tubes; Lancet; Sterile gauze pad; Povidone-iodine; 2 70% isopropyl alcohol prep pads; 10-mL red-top evacuated tube; Ice; Cup or emesis basin; Needle disposal unit; Biohazard bag

Discussion

Arterial blood gas measurements (ABGs) are used to evaluate gas exchange in the lungs by measuring the partial pressure of oxygen and carbon dioxide. Routine arterial puncture differs from routine venipuncture as follows:

1. **Patient preparation**: Collection of blood for ABG analysis is more painful for the patient than a routine venipuncture. Informing the patient of this before the procedure can lessen patient anxiety and promote patient cooperation, which is critical to the success of the operation. Many facilities have delegated the task of obtaining and analyzing blood gas specimens to the respiratory therapy department. Some facilities may require documentation of the specific type of respiratory therapy a patient is receiving prior to the collection of a specimen for ABG analysis. This is an additional rationale for respiratory therapists to collect ABGs instead of laboratory personnel.
2. **Equipment**: The equipment required for the collection of ABG specimens is as follows: a syringe that is impermeable to gas exchange; rubber stopper; heparin; 20- and 23-gauge needles; basin or plastic bag used to hold the ice and specimen during transport; and crushed ice.
3. **Preparation of equipment**: The syringe must be prepared before the collection of the arterial blood gas specimen. The plunger should be moved back and forth in the barrel of the syringe to ensure its mobility. After the plunger has been prepared, the syringe must be coated with heparin. The 20-gauge needle is attached to the syringe. The needle is used to puncture the stopper of the heparin vile. The plunger is pulled back and rotated until approximately 1.0 mL of heparin is introduced into the syringe. The needle is withdrawn from the stopper of the heparin vial. The syringe is "rolled" between the phlebotomist's hands to ensure complete coating of the syringe with the heparin. After the syringe has been coated with heparin, the excess heparin is expelled and the 20-gauge needle is removed. The 23-gauge needle is then aseptically attached and is used to collect the arterial blood gas specimen.

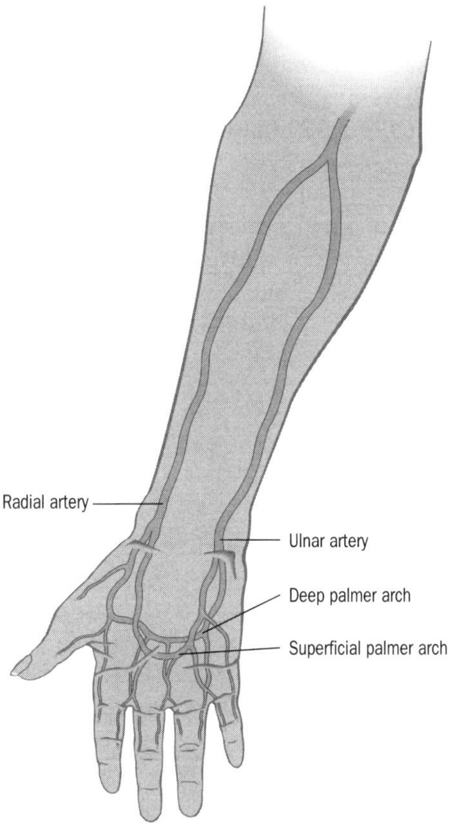

Figure 23-1 Arteries of the arm and hand.

4. **Positioning of the puncture site**: The puncture site of choice is the radial artery, which is located in the patient's wrist. The wrist should be supported with a rolled towel.

5. **Site selection**: Prior to selecting the specific site for arterial puncture, the patient's collateral circulation must be assessed by the Allen Test. If the Allen Test is abnormal, the phlebotomist must select another site for arterial blood sample collection. If the Allen Test is normal, the phlebotomist may collect blood from the radial artery. To locate this artery, use the index finger and middle finger to press down on the area where the artery is located (**Fig. 23-1**). The radial artery can be recognized by its pulsing. A tourniquet is NEVER used to assist in locating the radial artery.

6. **Site preparation**: Arterial puncture sites are cleansed using both alcohol and iodine. The iodine solution is applied to the puncture site first, followed by the alcohol. The site is then allowed to air dry. The phlebotomist's fingers are then cleaned in the same manner so that the site can be repalpated before collecting the arterial specimen.

7. **Location of the artery**: The artery is located by pressing down on the selected puncture site with one hand and holding the syringe in the other.

8. **Angle**: The needle should be inserted, bevel up, at a 45- to 60-degree angle.

9. **Depth**: Once the needle has pierced the vessel wall of the artery, the pulsation of the artery will force blood into the syringe. The syringe is allowed to fill with the pressure of the artery, forcing the blood into the syringe. Do NOT pull back on the plunger.

10. **Postpuncture care**: After collection of the blood specimen, pressure is applied to the puncture site for at least 5 minutes.

11. **Needle disposal**: The needle is not removed from the syringe for disposal. The needle is capped or stoppered using a single-handed method so that it is airtight.

12. **Specimen transport**: Specimens for ABG analysis are transported on ice.

Collecting arterial blood gases by arterial puncture is potentially a more dangerous procedure than venipuncture. Although potential complications exist with any invasive procedure, the complications associated with arterial puncture may be more serious than those associated with venipuncture. Three of the most common hazards associated with arterial puncture are hematoma, arteriospasm, and thrombosis.

Because arteries have more pressure exerted on them by the heart (as compared to veins), leakage of blood into the surrounding tissue after arterial puncture may occur at a faster rate than after venipuncture. To prevent hematoma following arterial puncture, pressure must be applied to the puncture site for at least 5 minutes. Patients who are taking anticoagulants, who have liver disease, or who are elderly may require a longer application of pressure.

Arteriospasm is a sudden, transient constriction of the artery, which may be a response to pain or other nervous stimuli. When arteriospasm occurs during arterial puncture, the artery is shut down, and blood collection may be impossible. Arteriospasm may also result in temporarily impaired blood supply to the tissue served by the artery.

A thrombus may form on the inner wall of a blood vessel after injury to that vessel. Thrombi usually form over time when a needle has been left in place; they rarely form after a single arterial puncture. Thrombi may occur in both arteries and veins, but they have more serious consequences in arteries because not all arteries have collateral vessels to provide adequate alternate blood supply. Thus, the safety of a particular site for arterial puncture primarily depends on the presence of collateral vessels.

Only those extensively trained and approved by the medical staff at a particular facility are allowed to perform arterial blood gases. For this reason, students will perform the Allen Test and site preparation only. Students will not practice arterial punctures on each other during the student lab.

The Allen Test

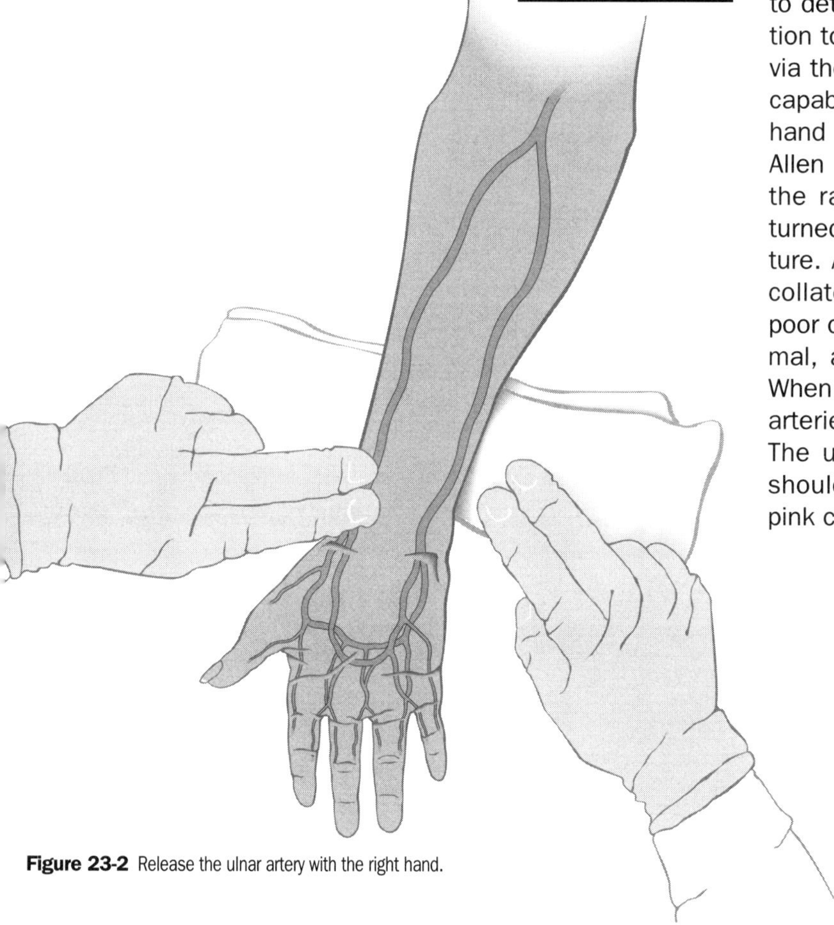

Figure 23-2 Release the ulnar artery with the right hand.

The Allen Test is performed prior to arterial puncture to determine if the patient has adequate collateral circulation to the hand. Oxygenated blood is supplied to the hand via the radial and ulnar arteries. During the Allen Test, the capability of the ulnar artery to provide circulation to the hand is measured by a color change. If the results of the Allen Test are normal, the radial artery (located medial to the radius bone and superficial to it when the hand is turned palm side up) is a suitable site for arterial puncture. An abnormal Allen Test result may indicate a lack of collateral circulation to the hand via the ulnar artery or poor coronary output. If results of the Allen Test are abnormal, another site for arterial puncture must be selected. When performing the Allen Test, both the radial and ulnar arteries are compressed while the patient makes a fist. The ulnar artery is then released (**Fig. 23-2**). The hand should turn pink within 5 seconds. Failure to restore a pink color within 5 seconds is an abnormal result.

Capillary Blood Gases

Capillary blood gases instead of arterial blood gases may be collected from infants and children. Arterial blood gas sampling may be too dangerous in infant and pediatric populations. The phlebotomist should follow standard procedures for site selection and patient preparation prior to capillary blood gas sampling. In addition, the following procedures must be followed:

1. The site must be warmed. Blood collected after skin puncture is a composition of arterial, venous, and capillary blood. When a skin puncture site is warmed, blood flow to the site is increased. The fraction of blood increased most significantly by warming the site is the arterial portion. Therefore, when a site is being prepared prior to the collection of capillary blood gases, it is necessary to warm the site to arterialize the specimen. Commercially prepared heel warmers or towels saturated with warm water (39–42°C) will accomplish this equally well. Warming the site may increase blood flow to the site up to sevenfold, which facilitates specimen collection. The increase is mostly on the arterial side of the circulation (rather than the venous side). Consequently, the sample obtained will be more arterial than venous in nature.

2. A metal filing (called a "flea") may be added to the collection tube prior to the collection of patient specimen to assist in mixing the specimen after collection (**Fig. 23-3**).

3. A heparinized capillary tube is used to collect the specimen.

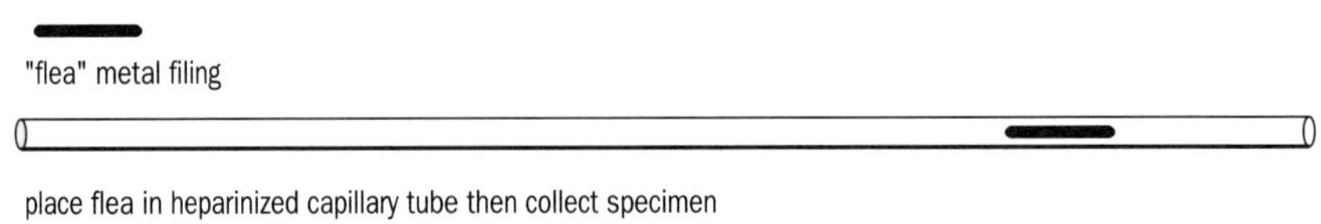

Figure 23-3 The metal filing, or "flea," used for mixing the specimen.

4. The specimen CANNOT be contaminated with air bubbles! Air in the specimen will result in significant changes in the oxygen partial pressure (PO_2) levels of the specimen when mixing.

5. After collection of the specimen, BOTH ends of the collection tube must be sealed with caps or sealing clay to prevent contamination of the specimen with air (**Fig. 23-4**).

6. A magnet is slid around the collection tube and moved up and down the tube. The magnet will cause the "flea" to move up and down inside the tube, mixing the specimen (**Fig. 23-4**).

7. The specimen should be appropriately labeled and transported on ice.

There are conflicting reports in the literature on the validity of PO_2 analysis performed on arterialized skin puncture specimens compared to arterial PO_2 analysis. Although one of the studies reported a clinically useful correlation over a narrow range of arterial PO_2 values under significant limitations of the technique, it was concluded that arterial specimens are preferred for blood gas analysis.

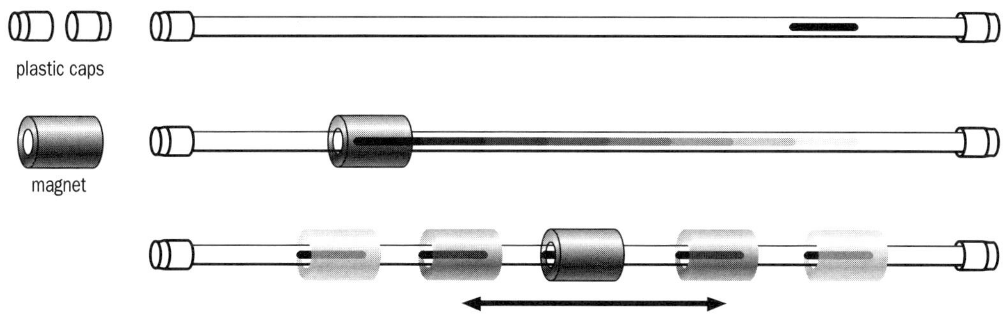

Figure 23-4 The tube is sealed with the plastic caps. Then the magnet is placed around the tube and moved up and down, causing the flea to move up and down inside the tube.

Because blood obtained by skin puncture is a mixture, the PO_2 would be expected to be lower in skin puncture blood than in arterial blood. The difference is greatest with high arterial PO_2 and with low blood flow. In newborn infants with anatomically patent ductus arteriosus and foramen ovale, crying may cause a functional right-to-left shunt, thus lowering the arterial PO_2, particularly in the domain of the descending aorta. Heel puncture blood from newborns, therefore, does not provide accurate results for the evaluation of oxygen tension.

Procedure 1: Allen Test

1. Approach the patient.
2. Identify the patient following standard identification procedures.
3. Explain the Allen Test procedure to the patient.
4. Rest the patient's arm on a bedside table, supporting the patient's wrist with a rolled towel.
5. Instruct the patient to clench his/her fist.
6. Using the middle and index finger of each hand, exert pressure on the radial and ulnar arteries simultaneously.
7. Instruct the patient to open his/her fist. Note the blanched color of the patient's palm, caused by impaired blood flow through both the ulnar and radial arteries.
8. Release the pressure on the ulnar artery. Maintain pressure on the radial artery (see **Fig. 23-2**).
9. Observe the patient's fist. If the palm returns to a normal color (pink) within 5 seconds, the Allen Test is normal. The radial artery may then be selected as a site for arterial puncture.

Procedure 2:

Site Preparation Prior to Arterial Puncture

1. Wash hands. Don gloves and gown.
2. Role play: Explain the arterial puncture procedure to the patient. Be honest. Explain that the procedure may be uncomfortable and more painful than a routine venipuncture. Be sure the patient understands that his/her cooperation is necessary to the success of the procedure.
3. Locate the radial artery (see **Fig. 23-1**). Arteries are located by exerting constant pressure in the general area an artery is routinely found. Do NOT palpate to locate an artery!
4. Cleanse the selected site with a povidone-iodine solution. Begin at the puncture site and move the applicator in concentric circles out from the site.
5. Cleanse your gloved fingers in the same manner.
6. Wipe the puncture site with alcohol. Cleanse your gloved fingers with alcohol.
7. Allow the puncture site to air dry.

REMINDER

Students are not allowed to perform arterial punctures on other students! This procedure ends with completion of site preparation.

Procedure 3:

Collection of Capillary Blood for Arterial Blood Gas Determinations

1. Wash hands. Don gloves and gown.
2. Approach the patient.
3. Identify the patient. Explain the procedure.
4. Apply commercially prepared heel warmer (or towel saturated with warm water) onto the site for 5 to 10 minutes.
5. Remove alcohol prep pad from the package. Place metal filing ("flea") in each specimen tube.
6. Cleanse the puncture site, using a circular motion.
7. Allow the site to air dry.
8. Hold the site securely.
9. Position the lancet above the puncture site.
10. Puncture the site selected.
11. Squeeze the site to produce a drop of blood at the puncture site.

12. Wipe the first drop of blood from the puncture site, using sterile gauze.
13. Collect 3 large-bore capillary tubes. Avoid air bubbles in the tubes.
14. Once the sample is collected, apply gauze to the puncture site.
15. Seal both ends of the specimen tubes.
16. Slip a magnet ring around each tube and invert several times. Remove the stopper from the 10-mL red-top evacuated tube. Place the sealed, large-bore capillary tubes in the evacuated tube (refer to Lab #14).
17. Appropriately label specimens. Submerge in an ice bath for transport.
18. Discard trash in the appropriate waste receptacles.

Checklist:

Allen Test/ Preparation of Site Prior to Arterial Puncture

Comments:

(A) Performed **(B) Needs Improvement** **(C) Not Performed**

_____1. Washes hands. Dons gloves and gown.
_____2. Role play: Identifies patient.
_____3. Role play: Approaches patient. Explains procedure to the patient, addressing the potential level of discomfort and stressing that patient cooperation is necessary for the success of the procedure.
_____4. Positions patient's wrist. Instructs patient to clench his/her fist.
_____5. Appropriately exerts pressure on the radial and ulnar arteries.
_____6. Instructs patient to open his/her fist.
_____7. Observes color of patient's hand.
_____8. Releases ulnar artery.
_____9. Observes color of patient's hand.
_____10. Correctly interprets the results of the Allen Test.
_____11. Locates the radial artery.
_____12. Appropriately cleanses the site, using povidone-iodine.
_____13. Appropriately cleanses gloved fingers.
_____14. Appropriately cleanses site and gloved fingers with alcohol.
_____15. Allows puncture site to air dry.

Checklist:

Collection of Capillary Blood Gases

Comments:

(A) Performed **(B) Needs Improvement** **(C) Not Performed**

______1. Washes hands. Dons gloves and gown.
______2. Role play: Approaches patient.
______3. Role play: Identifies patient, using 2-step method of patient identification.
______4. Role play: Explains procedure.
______5. Selects, prepares, and organizes equipment. Places the metal mixing bar (flea) in the specimen collection tubes.
______6. Selects site for skin puncture.
______7. Applies heel warmer to site for at least 5 minutes.
______8. Cleanses skin puncture site with alcohol.
______9. Allows site to air dry.
______10. Secures puncture site appropriately.
______11. Punctures site with lancet at correct angle.
______12. Wipes away the first drop of blood.
______13. Holds collection tube horizontal—or just below horizontal—to fill.
______14. Fills tube to the appropriate level.
______15. Fills tube without introducing air bubbles.
______16. Provides patient with gauze and instructs patient to apply pressure to the puncture site.
______17. Seals both ends of the tube.
______18. Slips magnet around collection bar and tips the tube back and forth to mix the specimen.
______19. Appropriately labels specimen.
______20. Prepares specimen for transport by submerging in ice.
______21. Checks puncture site to be sure bleeding has stopped.
______22. Discards lancet in the needle disposal unit.
______23. Removes equipment. Discards materials contaminated with blood in the biohazard bag.
______24. Appropriately discards other waste material.

Study Questions
Lab 23

1. Define collateral circulation. How does this term apply to blood circulation to the hand? ______________________________

____

2. Which blood specimen is preferable for ABG analysis: arterial or capillary? Why?

____

3. What effect will air bubbles have on a specimen collected for ABG analysis?

____

4. Why is ABG analysis often performed in the respiratory therapy department instead of the chemistry department of the laboratory? ______________________________

____

5. Define PO_2, PCO_2, pH. How are they related to arterial blood gas analysis?

____

6. How soon must a specimen for arterial blood gas analysis be delivered to the lab following collection? ______________________________

____

7. Why is the thumb NOT used to palpate for an artery prior to arterial blood sampling? ______________________________

____

8. Compare and contrast arterial puncture and venipuncture, from the patient's point of view. ______________________________

____

LAB 24

Preparation of Blood Smears for Malarial Screening

Objective

To introduce the procedure associated with the preparation of smears to be used for malarial screening procedures; to gain expertise in routine blood film preparation; to gain expertise in performing skin punctures

Equipment

Gloves; Gown; 70% isopropyl alcohol prep pad; Sterile gauze; Sterile lancet; 8 glass slides; Needle disposal unit; Biohazard bag

Discussion

Malaria is usually caused by 1 of 4 species of the protozoan *Plasmodium*: *P. vivax, P. falciparum, P. malariae,* or *P. ovale.* The parasites may be transferred to humans by infected female Anopheles mosquitoes, via infected blood transfusions, through sharing contaminated needles, and congenitally. Humans act as host to the malarial parasite for the asexual portion of its life cycle. The parasites may be detected in the infected patient's bloodstream through the examination of peripheral blood films stained with Giemsa stain. Identification of the species causing the infection is important to successfully treat the patient.

Symptoms in persons with malaria will vary, based on what species is causing the infection. The symptom common to all persons infected with a species of *Plasmodium,* however, is fever. Geographic regions considered endemic for malaria include Africa, Korea, certain sections of the South Pacific, and Vietnam.

Blood smears for malarial screen are usually collected from patients at 6- to 8-hour intervals for at least 3 successive days to increase the likelihood of recovering the parasites. Specimen collection for malarial screen does not have to coincide with episodes of chills and fever in the patient. Unlike bacteremia, fever spikes do not characteristically coincide with release of the parasite into the bloodstream. Specimens for malarial screen may be collected directly from the patient's finger, following skin puncture procedures. It is also appropriate to collect an EDTA tube by venipuncture and prepare the smears from blood aliquoted from the EDTA tube.

Screening techniques for malarial parasites in a patient's bloodstream incorporate the use of 2 thick and 2 thin smears. The smears are stained with Giemsa stain and examined microscopically. Thick smears are used to screen for the presence of malarial parasites in the blood. Thin smears are used to identify the species of parasite causing the infection.

Procedure 1: Thick Film Preparation

1. Place 1 large drop of blood on a glass slide (**Fig. 24-1**).
2. Using the corner of a second slide, spread the drop of blood on the slide until it approximates the size of a dime (**Fig. 24-2**, **Fig. 24-3**).
3. Prepare 3 films in this manner.
4. Label the 3 thick films.
5. Allow to air dry (approximately 30 minutes).

Procedure 2: Thin Film Preparation

1. Follow standard procedures for thin film preparation (refer to **Figs. 12-1, 12-2,** and **12-3**).
2. Prepare 3 thin films.
3. Label the 3 thin films.
4. Allow to air dry.

Figure 24-1 Top and side view of relative size and placement of a drop of blood for thick smear.

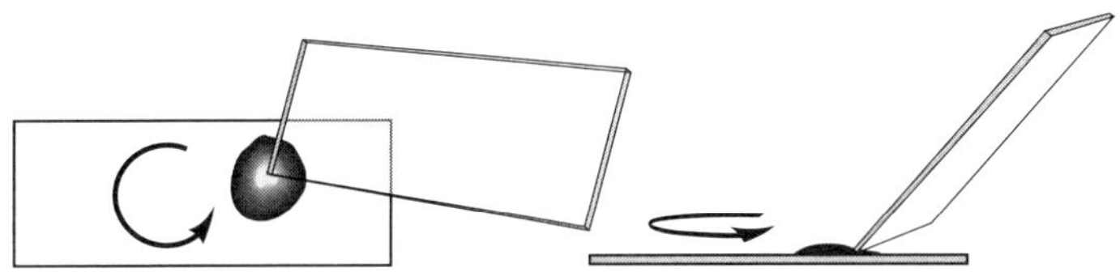

Figure 24-2 Top and side view of the positioning of spreader slide to prepare a thick smear for malarial screen.

Figure 24-3 Top and side view of a thick smear for malarial screen.

Assignment

Perform a skin puncture on your lab partner. Using the blood obtained, prepare 6 smears appropriate for malarial screening procedures. Present the smears to your instructor for evaluation.

Comments:

Checklist: Thick Smears

(A) Performed **(B) Needs Improvement** **(C) Not Performed**

_____ _____ _____1. Approximates the thickness of the thick portion of a smear prepared by the slide/wedge procedure.
_____ _____ _____2. Is circular, approximating the size of a dime.
_____ _____ _____3. Is appropriately labeled.

Comments:

Checklist: Thin Smears

(A) Performed **(B) Needs Improvement** **(C) Not Performed**

_____ _____ _____1. Has a smooth, even surface.
_____ _____ _____2. Has a thick portion, which tapers off into a thinner portion.
_____ _____ _____3. Ends in a feathered edge.
_____ _____ _____4. Covers one half to two thirds of the slide.
_____ _____ _____5. Has an appropriate thickness (is neither too thick nor too thin).
_____ _____ _____6. Has a space on either side of the smear.
_____ _____ _____7. Is appropriately labeled.

Study Questions

Lab 24

1. What is the difference between Giemsa stain and Wright's stain? When is each used? ______

2. Which of the 4 malarial protozoans is recovered most frequently? Which of the 4 protozoans is associated with the most deadly form of malaria?

3. How is malaria related to sickle cell anemia? ______

4. How often would you expect blood smears for malarial screening ordered at your facility? ______

5. What types of medications are used to prevent and/or treat malaria?

LAB 25

Blood Donor Workups

Objective

To introduce the following procedures of blood donor workups: medical history screening; physical assessment of the donor; preparation of the venipuncture site prior to the collection of a unit of blood; and postdonation care

Equipment

Donor record card; Scale; Thermometer; Sphygmomanometer; Stethoscope; 70% isopropyl alcohol prep pads; Sterile gauze; Blood lancet; Gloves; Gown; 2 capillary tubes; Donor site prep kit; Adhesive bandages; Donor bags (for demonstration purposes only); Needle disposal unit; Biohazard bag

Discussion

When collecting a unit of blood from a donor, the phlebotomist must follow certain procedures to ensure the safety of the donor during the donation process. In addition, the phlebotomist must adhere to certain standards in order to collect a quality unit of blood or blood product. The standards have been established by the American Association of Blood Banks to provide the safest possible transfusion to the patient.

AIDS

According to the AABB *Standards for Blood Banks and Transfusion Services*, all donors must be given educational materials informing them of activities that place them at high risk for HIV infection. Persons at risk for HIV infection must refrain from donating blood. Donor screening must include questions relating to the signs and symptoms of AIDS, including evidence of HIV infection, AIDS-related complex (ARC), and Kaposi's sarcoma. Answers suggestive of disease must be evaluated for determination of donor suitability. Potential donors who, since 1977, have migrated from or been a resident in those non–U.S. locations identified on the current Food and Drug Administration (FDA) listing of areas with increased risk of HIV-1 and HIV-2 transmission will be deferred indefinitely.

Many facilities provide information sheets for blood donors, which emphasize that blood should not be donated by persons wanting to ensure that they do not have AIDS (ie, a person should not donate blood to receive a "free" AIDS test). Donors who may be at risk for AIDS may confidentially self-exclude their blood from the general blood supply. Following is an example of a blood donor information sheet used by Christ Hospital and Medical Center, Oak Lawn, IL.

Information for all Blood Donors

YOU MUST NOT DONATE BLOOD TO RECEIVE AN AIDS TEST...WHY NOT?

- If you are or have been at risk of catching or spreading the AIDS virus, you may have the virus in your blood, yet feel completely healthy.
- No test currently available can detect all infectious blood. There is an interval during the early stage of infection when the HIV-1 antibody test may be negative; however, the infection may still be transmitted.
- If you donate anyway, you could infect the patient(s) who receive your blood components. Your blood donation may further endanger the life of a sick or injured person.
- If you want to be tested for HIV-1 or are at risk of transmitting AIDS, there is an easier, safer, and faster alternative.
- Your doctor or local health department can provide information about confidential testing locations and/or counseling services. It takes just a phone call. You need not identify yourself.

TESTING PROCEDURES

If your unit of blood is found to be HIV-1 antibody positive, it will not be used for transfusion. If the test results are confirmed using a more specific test, you will be notified according to Christ Hospital and Medical Center standard policy; however, in the case of HIV, notification may be delayed up to 6 weeks. Testing at public health clinics is available much quicker and your name will not become part of a donor deferral registry. Names of blood donors with confirmed positive results will be included on a list of permanently deferred donors who are no longer eligible to donate blood.

Your blood will be tested for the following disease indicators:

Hepatitis B—HBsAg	Hepatitis B core antibody—HBc
Hepatitis C—HCV (previously called non-A, non-B)	AIDS—HIV-1 Human T-lymphotropic virus type I—HTLV-I
Syphilis—RPR	ALT, a liver enzyme, and other viruses and retroviruses

PLEASE HELP US ENSURE A SAFE BLOOD SUPPLY

- In many circumstances, a donor may not feel comfortable deferring before the actual donation of blood has occurred.
- If after donating blood, you realize that you should not have donated because of previous risk factors, behaviors, or diseases, your blood must NOT be used for transfusion.
- Call Christ Hospital and Medical Center Blood Bank within 24 hours after your donation, and ask that your blood not be used for transfusion. The only information that you will need to give is the Unit Identification Number and the date of your donation.

CONFIDENTIALITY WILL BE MAINTAINED AT ALL TIMES IN ACCORDANCE WITH STATE LAW.

NOTIFICATION OF POSITIVE TEST RESULTS

If your blood test results are confirmed positive for any of the following tests, it will not be transfused to a patient and you will be notified in accordance with Christ Hospital and Medical Center established policy and applicable state laws:

HIV (human immunodeficiency virus)—AIDS virus	HBsAg (hepatitis B antigen)—hepatitis B
HTLV-I (human T-lymphotropic virus type I)—associated with T-cell leukemia and tropical spastic paraparesis	HCV (hepatitis C antibody)—hepatitis C Abnormal level ALT (alanine aminotransferase)—elevated liver enzyme
Syphilis	Other viruses or retroviruses

Medical History Screening

Prospective donors are asked a series of questions related to their medical history. Usually, blood donation centers have the questions listed on a card or form. Following is an example of the medical history question section from the blood donor registration card used by Christ Hospital and Medical Center, Oak Lawn, IL.

NOTE TO BLOOD DONORS: Please answer the following questions as truthfully and honestly as possible. We need to know if you have or have had any of these in your medical history.

1. When did you eat last?______________________
2. When did you last have alcohol?________________

Yes/No

- ❑ ❑ 3. Have you donated blood under another name at this blood center? Have you been rejected as a donor?
- ❑ ❑ 4. Are you feeling well today?
- ❑ ❑ 5. Have you donated blood in the last 8 weeks? Platelets within 48 hours?
- ❑ ❑ 6. Are you pregnant? Have you been pregnant in the last six weeks?
- ❑ ❑ 7. Have you had any surgery, hospitalization or serious illness in the last year?
- ❑ ❑ 8. Have you ever had tuberculosis, shortness of breath, swollen ankles, chest pain, disease of the heart, lungs, kidneys, liver, or stomach?
- ❑ ❑ 9. Have you had any unexplained weight loss recently? How much?
- ❑ ❑ 10. Have you taken any drugs or medicine within the last 2 weeks? Any aspirin in the last 5 days?
- ❑ ❑ 11. Had fainting spells, convulsions, or epilepsy?
- ❑ ❑ 12. Have you bled long when cut or tooth pulled? Had leukemia, polycythemia, or other blood disease?
- ❑ ❑ 13. Had a tooth extraction or oral surgery in the last 3 days?
- ❑ ❑ 14. Have you diabetes requiring insulin treatment?
- ❑ ❑ 15. Do you have any cold or respiratory problems?

Yes/No

- ❑ ❑ 16. Do you have any skin infections, boils, or open wounds?
- ❑ ❑ 17. Were you born in or did you move to the U.S. from a part of Africa south of the Sahara Desert or islands close to that part of Africa?
- ❑ ❑ 18. Have you at any time since 1977 engaged in sex for money or drugs?
- ❑ ❑ 19. Have you even one time since 1977
  Men: Had sexual contact with another man?
  Women: Had sexual contact with a man who has had sex with another man?
- ❑ ❑ 20. Have you used IV drugs even one time or been addicted to drugs or alcohol?
- ❑ ❑ 21. Had a positive HIV antibody test (AIDS)?
- ❑ ❑ 22. Have you been diagnosed as having AIDS or AIDS-related complex (ARC)?
- ❑ ❑ 23. Have you received factor VIII (AHF), factor IX, or clotting factor concentrates?
- ❑ ❑ 24. Have you any unexplained fevers, night sweats, persistent cough, persistent diarrhea, greatly enlarged lymph nodes in your neck, underarms, or groin areas, any bluish/purple spots on or under your skin or mucosa membranes or noticed any white patches in your mouth?
- ❑ ❑ 25. Did you serve in the military or as a civilian during the Persian Gulf War of 1991?

Yes/No

❑ ❑ 26. Have you engaged in sex with a person who has: hemophilia, received factor VIII, factor IX, or other clotting factors; used IV drugs, a diagnosis of AIDS, ARC, AIDS symptoms, or a positive HIV test?

❑ ❑ 27. In the past 2 weeks have you been vaccinated for measles (rubeola), mumps, polio (oral), smallpox, yellow fever, or with any animal serum products?

❑ ❑ 28. In the past 4 weeks have you been vaccinated for German measles (rubella)? Have you taken Accutane?

❑ ❑ 29. In the past six months have you visited a malarial area?

IN THE PAST YEAR HAVE YOU:

❑ ❑ 30. Had your ears pierced? Had tattoos? Had acupuncture? Had an accidental needlestick?

❑ ❑ 31. Lived with someone who has had hepatitis? Lived in a prison or mental hospital? Worked where hepatitis is endemic?

❑ ❑ 32. Had hepatitis B immune globulin or any unlicensed vaccines? Rabies injections? Blood group immunization?

❑ ❑ 33. Had a sexually transmitted disease? Syphilis? Gonorrhea? Been sexually assaulted?

Yes/No

❑ ❑ 34. Engaged in sex with a man or woman who receives drugs or money for such activity?

❑ ❑ 35. Received a blood transfusion or any blood components?

IN THE PAST 3 YEARS HAVE YOU:

❑ ❑ 36. Had malaria, lived in a malarial area, or taken medication for malaria?

❑ ❑ 37. Taken the medication Tegison?

PERMANENT DEFERRAL—HAVE YOU EVER:

❑ ❑ 38. Had hepatitis or yellow jaundice (after 10 years of age), or a positive test for hepatitis (HBsAg), hepatitis C?

❑ ❑ 39. Had an injection of PIT-HgH (pituitary human growth hormone)?

❑ ❑ 40. Had a history of babesiosis or Chagas' disease?

❑ ❑ 41. I have read, understood, and had the opportunity to answer questions regarding the educational literature provided by the blood bank concerning AIDS and understand that members of groups at increased risk have been asked to refrain from donating at this time. I believe that my blood is safe for transfusion and have answered the above questions accurately to the best of my knowledge.

I have reviewed and understand the donor eligibility information and the blood donation process. I agree NOT to donate blood or plasma for transfusion to another person or for further manufacture if I have AIDS, a positive HIV antibody test, or if any of the activities or signs and symptoms associated with AIDS apply to me. I understand that my blood will be tested for laboratory evidence of infectious agents capable of transmission through blood transfusion including, but not limited to, the AIDS virus, hepatitis B, and other viruses. I understand that I will be notified of test results that are important to my health and may affect my eligibility to be a blood donor. If my HIV, hepatitis, or other test results are confirmed positive my blood will not be transfused and my name will become part of a list of permanently deferred blood donors. I understand that test results and medical history information will not be released without my written consent, except as required by law. I have truthfully answered all medical questions. I am voluntarily donating my blood to be used as determined by Christ Hospital and Medical Center, and I at my own risk, for good consideration, hereby release Christ Hospital and Medical Center and its staff from all claims and demands incidental to or relative to the donation of this blood.

Signature of Donor:________________________ Date:__________ Interviewed by:____________________

The donor's responses to the questions are recorded, and the card is signed by the donor to verify the information provided. Donors may be deferred permanently or temporarily, based on their medical history. The following chart lists conditions that may cause a donor to be deferred. Conditions resulting in permanent donor deferral are listed first, followed by conditions resulting in temporary donor deferral.

Conditions That May Permanently Defer a Donor

Condition
AIDS
Chronic kidney disease
Convulsions or fainting spells after infancy
Diabetes controlled by insulin
Donation of the only unit of blood transfused to a patient who developed hepatitis within 6 months of the transfusion
Epilepsy, convulsions
Heart disease, liver disease, lung disease, cancer, abnormal bleeding tendency (subject to evaluation by a physician)
History of intravenous drug abuse
Open heart surgery
Positive hepatitis B surface antigen test
Viral hepatitis infection after age 10

Conditions That May Temporarily Defer a Donor

Condition	Length of Deferral
Active allergies	Until free of symptoms
Acute cough, sore throat, cold	Until free of symptoms
Age	Persons must be 17 years of age or older to donate blood
Antibiotics (oral)	None if for dermatology, otherwise depends on condition
Asthma	6 months after last attack
Blood transfusion	1 year after transfusion
Close contact with a hepatitis patient	6 months
Drug therapy, including antibiotics, anticoagulants, digitalis, insulin, anticonvulsants, vasodilators, antiarrythmics	Clinical condition for such treatment may defer a donor
Ear piercing/Tattooing/Acupuncture	6 months
Former inmates of penal institutions	6 months
German measles (rubella)	4 weeks
History of malaria or a history of antimalarial prophylaxis or residents of countries endemic for malaria	3 years after becoming asymptomatic or discontinuing therapy
Inoculation with attenuated virus, including: polio (oral), measles (rubeola), mumps, yellow fever	2 weeks
Major surgery/illness	6 months
Malarial area (no medication)	6 months (assuming donor has been free of unexplained febrile episodes and has not taken antimalarial drugs)
Malarial area (with medication)	3 years after completing drug
Minor surgery	After healing is complete
Miscarriage	6 weeks
Mononucleosis	6 months after becoming asymptomatic
Pregnancy	Duration of pregnancy and 6 weeks following conclusion of the pregnancy
Rabies (duck embryo or human diploid)	No deferral, unless the episode followed the bite of a rabid animal, in which case the prospective donor is deferred for 12 months
Recent blood donation	8 weeks (there must be an 8-week interval between blood donations)
Recipient of blood or blood products	6 months
Recipients of hepatitis B immunoglobulin (HBIG)	12 months
Skin cancer	1 month
Smallpox	Until scab has fallen off, or 2 weeks after immune reaction
Tooth extraction	72 hours if not on antibiotics
Tuberculosis	Until condition is successfully treated and no longer active
Unexplained recent weight loss of 10 lbs or more	Until physician has evaluated the potential donor and approved participation as a blood donor
Vaccinations; inoculation with toxoids and killed virus, bacterial and rickettsial vaccines, including hepatitis B, diphtheria, pertussis, typhoid, paratyphoid, cholera, typhus, Rocky Mountain spotted fever, influenza, polio (injection), plague	No deferral if prospective donor is symptom-free and afebrile
Weight	Persons must weigh over 110 lbs to donate blood

Physical Assessment of the Prospective Donor

Following the interview to determine a prospective donor's medical history, the phlebotomist must obtain certain measurements to ensure the donor falls within acceptable parameters. These measurements include weight, temperature, blood pressure, pulse, hemoglobin or hematocrit screening, evaluation of venipuncture site, and evaluation of the general appearance of the donor.

1. **Weight**: For the routine collection of a unit of blood from a donor, the donor must weigh at least 110 lbs (50 kg). If a prospective donor weighs less than this, the removal of a standard unit of blood may alter the donor's blood volume by too great a margin, which may result in an adverse donor reaction. If donor room personnel suspect a prospective donor does not meet the minimum weight requirement, the prospective donor should be weighed for an accurate assessment.
2. **Temperature**: The prospective donor must not have a temperature exceeding 37.5°C (99.5°F). Each donor's temperature is measured using an oral thermometer prior to blood donation.
3. **Blood pressure**: A sphygmomanometer (blood pressure cuff) is the instrument used to measure arterial blood pressure. The sphygmomanometer may be equipped with either a mercury manometer or an aneroid gauge. Both of these instruments are attached by rubber tubing to an inflatable rubber cuff. The donor's blood pressure is read off of one of these gauges to help determine the donor's eligibility. The systolic pressure should be no higher than 180 mm Hg, and the diastolic pressure should be no higher than 100 mm Hg.
4. **Pulse**: The prospective donor's pulse rate should be between 50 and 100 beats per minute. The pulse should be regular and steady, revealing no cardiac irregularity.
5. **Hemoglobin or hematocrit determinations**: Hemoglobin levels collected by fingerstick must be equal to or in excess of 12.5 g/dL to qualify a donor. Hematocrit levels collected by fingerstick must be equal to or in excess of 38% to qualify a donor.
6. **Examination of the venipuncture site**: The skin at the site selected for venipuncture must be free of lesions.
7. **General appearance of the donor**: The appearance of the donor should be consistent with good health. The donor should not be under the influence of drugs or alcohol.

Procedure 1: Donor History

1. Obtain a donor record card.
2. Fill in the donor's personal history, including name, address, and age.
3. Determine the donor's medical history by posing the questions listed on the donor record card to the donor.
4. If the donor answers "yes" to any of the questions asked, the interviewer must investigate further to determine the donor's eligibility. The donor's eligibility is based on the criteria presented in the discussion section of this lab. If the interviewer is unsure about a donor's eligibility, the interviewer should consult the blood bank supervisor and/or pathologist. Results of the additional investigation must appear as a note on the donor record card. For example, if the donor is asked, "Have you ever gotten a tattoo?" and the donor responds positively, the date the tattoo was obtained must be determined to evaluate the donor's eligibility.
5. The date of the donor's last donation must be recorded.
6. The date of the interview, the interviewer's initials, and the donor's signature must also be completed on the donor record card.

Procedure 2: Donor Physical

1. Weight: Determine the prospective donor's weight. Generally, the donor only needs to validate his/her weight if the donor appears to weigh less than 110 lbs.
2. Temperature: Take the donor's temperature by placing a thermometer under the patient's tongue. Allow the thermometer to remain in place long enough to obtain an accurate measurement. Many thermometers with digital readouts will sound an audio alarm when the donor's temperature has been accurately determined.
3. Blood Pressure
   A. Refer to Lab #4 for equipment quality control procedures.
   B. Have the donor sit in a comfortable position so the arm selected will

be slightly flexed and supported by a smooth, firm surface. The artery over which the blood pressure is to be recorded should be at the same level as the donor's heart. Blood pressure is decreased in a raised arm and increased in a lowered arm.

C. Be sure any residual air has been expelled from the cuff. Wrap the cuff around the patient's arm and position it so it rests 1 inch above the antecubital fossa. Be sure the tubes from the cuff do not rest over the brachial artery. Avoid clothing interference when positioning the blood pressure cuff. Placing the blood pressure cuff over bulky clothing may result in an uneven distribution of pressure. If a donor rolls his/her sleeve up too tightly, it may have the same effect as a tourniquet and affect pressure readings.
D. Using your fingertips, locate the brachial artery.
E. Using an alcohol prep pad, cleanse the ear pieces of the stethoscope. Dry with a piece of sterile gauze.
F. Place the bell of the stethoscope over the brachial artery. The bell of the stethoscope should not come in contact with the blood pressure cuff or with the patient's clothing, because this may alter the sounds for which the phlebotomist is listening, which may introduce an error into the blood pressure reading. Hold the bell of the stethoscope over the brachial artery so an airtight seal is created.
G. Place the earpieces angled forward in each of your ears.
H. Inflate the blood pressure cuff. Listen for the pulsation of the artery. Continue inflating the cuff until the pulsation of the artery is no longer heard. Be careful not to confuse body sounds with blood pressure sounds. Room noises may also interfere with the examiner's ability to hear blood pressure sounds.
I. Release the bulb of the cuff to allow the cuff to deflate at a rate of 2 to 3 mm Hg per heartbeat. Watch the mercury manometer or the aneroid

gauge as the cuff is deflated. If the cuff is deflated too rapidly, readings may be higher than the donor's true pressure. If a systolic or diastolic pressure is not obtained on the first attempt, the cuff should be entirely deflated and the reading taken again.

J. When the pulsation sound of the artery is heard again, the pressure of the aneroid gauge or mercury manometer is almost equal to the systolic pressure within the blood vessel. Note where the gauge pointed or where the column of mercury was located when the pulsation of the artery was heard. That point corresponds to the systolic reading.

K. Allow the blood pressure cuff to continue to deflate. The sounds will change from loud to soft, gradually diminishing until pulsation sounds are no longer detected. The location of the mercury on a mercury manometer or the needle on an aneroid gauge corresponding to the last, soft "thump" sound is the diastolic pressure.

L. Record the systolic/diastolic pressure on the donor's card.

4. Pulse

A. The donor should be sitting or lying down. The arm to be tested should be supported and relaxed.

B. Place the fingertips of the index, middle, and ring fingers over the donor's radial artery. NOTE: Never use the thumb to evaluate a donor's pulse. The thumb contains a pulse, which may be confused with the donor's pulse.

C. Exert pressure on the artery so the pulsation may be felt distinctly.

D. Count the pulse for exactly 60 seconds. The rate of the pulse must be accurately measured. The rate is recorded as number of beats per minute. The rhythm should also be evaluated. Normal rhythm is a regular beat, with the same amount of time lapse between each beat. In addition, the beats should be of the same strength. Variations in pulse rhythms should be evaluated by the donor's physician.

E. Record the pulse rate and rhythm on the donor's record card.

5. Hematocrit: Consult Lab #11 for procedural details. Determine the donor's hematocrit and record it on the donor's record card.
6. Evaluation of the venipuncture site: Look for signs of needle puncture marks, rashes, and any other suspect skin lesions in the antecubital fossa.
7. Evaluation of the donor's general appearance: The prospective donor should appear to be in good general health. The donor should NOT appear to be under the influence of drugs or alcohol or unduly nervous or apprehensive.

Procedure 3: Donor Phlebotomy

1. Identification
   A. Donor name.
   B. Donor identification number.
   C. Check the numbers assigned to the processing tubes attached to the donor bag. Be sure the numbers on the processing tubes identically match the numbers on the collection bag.
2. Site selection
   A. Apply a tourniquet to the donor's forearm or apply a blood pressure cuff inflated to between 40 and 60 mm Hg.
   B. Choose a large, firm vein in an area free of skin lesions, following routine procedures for vein selection prior to venipuncture.
   C. Loosen the tourniquet or deflate the blood pressure cuff.
3. Site preparation: Prepare the site prior to blood donation following aseptic technique. The site must be prepared 3 inches in diameter, using sterile materials and instruments.
   A. Scrub the puncture site 3 inches in diameter for 30 seconds using a .7% aqueous scrub solution of an iodophor compound. Remove excess foam.
   B. Apply iodophor-complex solution (10% PVP iodine) and let stand for 30 seconds.
   C. Cover area with sterile gauze.
   D. Do NOT repalpate the vein.

4. Venipuncture

A. Inspect the bag. Use a hemastat to clamp the tubing between the needle and the bag (**Fig. 25-1**).

B. Position the bag below the donor's arm.

C. Reapply the tourniquet or blood pressure cuff and have the donor pump his/her fist a few times.

D. Have the donor close the fist and hold it closed.

E. Unsheath the needle. Anchor the vein selected and insert the needle bevel up. Tape the needle and tubing to hold the needle in place.

F. Remove the clamp between the bag and the needle.

G. Have the donor periodically open and close the fist. This may be facilitated if a donor has something to squeeze, like a rubber ball or a rolled face towel.

H. Observe the donor throughout the donation.

I. Mix the blood with the anticoagulant in the bag by inverting the bag gently. Be sure the bag remains lower than the donor's arm. Repeat this several times during the donation process.

J. Collect a sufficient amount of blood. The acceptable weight range of donor units is 405 to 495 g.

K. When the donation is complete, clamp a hemastat on the tubing attached to the needle next to the bag.

L. Remove the tourniquet or blood pressure cuff and tape. Withdraw the needle and insert the needle through the stopper of the attached pilot evacuated tube.

M. Instruct the donor to apply pressure to the puncture site and elevate his/her arm—with the elbow straight—above his/her head.

N. Force the remaining blood in the tubing into the pilot evacuated tube. Seal the tubing using a heat sealer, next to the needle.

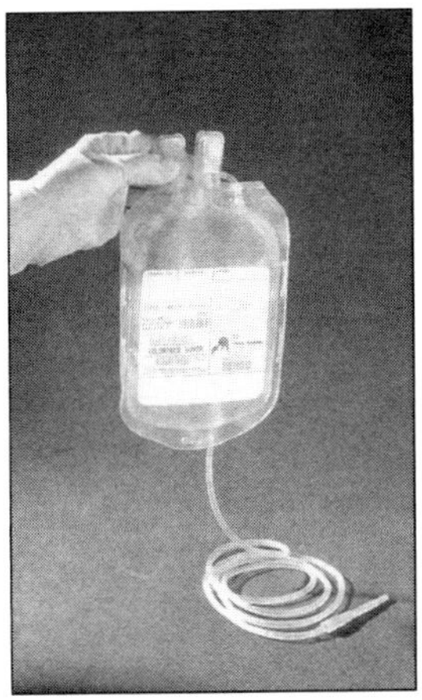

Figure 25-1 Donor blood bag.

O. Release the hemastat. The blood will automatically fill the tube. Force the blood from the tubing back into the donor bag at least 3 times. Heat-seal several sections. These sections will be used for crossmatching.

P. Fold the sections and secure through the loops on the side of the blood bag. Place the unit in the designated refrigerator.

Since the donor will provide between 405 and 495 mL of blood at one donation, the donor must be closely evaluated by donor room personnel before he/she is allowed to resume normal activities.

Procedure 4: Postphlebotomy Donor Care

1. Examine the donor's arm.
   A. If the site has stopped bleeding, fold a sterile gauze into quarters.
   B. Place the folded gauze over the puncture site.
   C. Apply the tape of a bandage on one side of the puncture site. Pull the bandage tightly over the gauze and secure on the opposite side of the puncture site.

2. Allow the donor to sit up when he/she feels and appears ready. When the donor feels ready, allow him/her to move to the observation area, where the donor should be offered something to eat and drink. If the donor feels or appears ill, administer first aid, as outlined in the "General Safety Guidelines" section of this workbook. Notify your instructor or supervisor.

3. Instruct the donor in postphlebotomy care.
   A. Increase fluids over the next 4 hours.
   B. No alcohol until after the donor has eaten.
   C. No smoking for at least one-half hour after donation.
   D. If the puncture site begins to bleed, the donor should raise his/her arm and apply pressure until the bleeding has stopped.
   E. Resume all normal activities within one-half hour of completion of donation if the donor feels well enough.

Checklist:

Blood Donor Workups

(A) Performed **(B) Needs Improvement** **(C) Not Performed**

Comments:

_____ 1. Appropriately takes donor history, using donor record card.
_____ 2. Correctly interprets donor history to accept or defer prospective donor.
_____ 3. Accurately determines patient's temperature.
_____ 4. Interprets patient's temperature to accept or defer donor.
_____ 5. Appropriately positions patient's arm for accurate blood pressure measurement.
_____ 6. Appropriately positions blood pressure cuff around patient's arm.
_____ 7. Locates brachial artery.
_____ 8. Appropriately places earpieces in ears. Appropriately places the bell of the stethoscope over the brachial artery.
_____ 9. Appropriately inflates blood pressure cuff.
_____ 10. Inflates blood pressure cuff to an appropriate level.
_____ 11. Appropriately deflates blood pressure cuff.
_____ 12. Deflates blood pressure cuff at an appropriate rate.
_____ 13. Obtains an accurate reading of the patient's blood pressure.
_____ 14. Correctly interprets blood pressure reading to accept or defer the prospective donor.
_____ 15. Appropriately locates patient's radial pulse.
_____ 16. Uses index and middle fingers to measure pulse rate and rhythm.
_____ 17. Accurately determines donor's pulse rate and rhythm.
_____ 18. Correctly interprets pulse rate and rhythm to accept or defer the prospective donor.
_____ 19. Washes hands. Dons gloves and gown.
_____ 20. Selects site for skin puncture.

Comments: **(A) Performed** **(B) Needs Improvement** **(C) Not Performed**

_____21. Gently massages donor's finger.
_____22. Removes alcohol prep pad from package.
_____23. Appropriately cleanses skin puncture site.
_____24. Allows site to air dry.
_____25. Holds patient's finger securely.
_____26. Positions lancet above skin puncture site.
_____27. Appropriately punctures site.
_____28. Squeezes finger to create a drop of blood at the puncture site.
_____29. Wipes off the first drop of blood.
_____30. Collects 2 capillary tubes.
_____31. Applies gauze to the skin puncture site once sample has been collected.
_____32. Seals the end of the capillary tubes with sealing clay.
_____33. Places the sealed capillary tubes in the microhematocrit centrifuge.
_____34. Positions the capillary tubes exactly opposite each other, the sealed ends pointing outward.
_____35. Centrifuges for an appropriate length of time. (Follows safety guidelines for centrifugation established at your facility.)
_____36. Reads the results using the microhematocrit tube reader.
_____37. Correctly interprets the results to accept or defer the donor.
_____38. Records the results on the donor record card.
_____39. Evaluates the venipuncture site; determines its appropriateness.
_____40. Evaluates the donor's general appearance; determines whether the donor's appearance is consistent with suitability for donation.
_____41. Checks the identification numbers on the pilot tubes and donor bag to ensure that the numbers match exactly.
_____42. Selects a site appropriate for donor phlebotomy.
_____43. Scrubs puncture site in 3-inch diameter.

Comments: **(A) Performed** **(B) Needs Improvement** **(C) Not Performed**

_____ 44. Scrubs puncture site for 30 seconds, using .7% aqueous scrub solution of an iodophor compound.
_____ 45. Removes excess foam.
_____ 46. Applies iodophor-complex solution (10% PVP iodine) and lets stand for 30 seconds.
_____ 47. Covers site with sterile gauze.
_____ 48. Clamps tubing between needle and bag.
_____ 49. Appropriately positions bag.
_____ 50. Reapplies tourniquet or blood pressure cuff.
_____ 51. Instructs donor to make a fist.
_____ 52. Appropriately performs venipuncture.
_____ 53. Unclamps hemastat between needle and bag.
_____ 54. Periodically mixes blood with anticoagulant.
_____ 55. Collects an acceptable amount of blood in the bag.
_____ 56. Removes the tourniquet or blood pressure cuff.
_____ 57. Removes tape.
_____ 58. Appropriately applies a hemastat.
_____ 59. Withdraws needle.
_____ 60. Instructs the donor to apply pressure at the puncture site and to elevate the arm over the head.
_____ 61. Forces blood from the tubing into the appropriate processing tube.
_____ 62. Removes clamp between the bag and the needle.
_____ 63. Forces blood from the tubing back into the blood bag several times.
_____ 64. Prepares segments by heat sealing the tubing in appropriate intervals.
_____ 65. Appropriately packages the tubing to store the unit.
_____ 66. Appropriately bandages donor's arm.
_____ 67. Appropriately instructs the donor in postdonation care.

Study Questions

Lab 25

1. Compare and contrast autologous blood donation and directed donation.

2. What is a therapeutic phlebotomy? With what condition is it most commonly associated?

3. Compare and contrast collection containers used following venipuncture and donor collection bags.

4. List and define at least 3 different preservatives used in blood donor bags.

5. What tests are routinely performed on a unit of blood before transfusion?

6. Compare and contrast potential complications of blood donation with potential complications of routine venipuncture.

LAB 26

Role Playing

Objective

To simulate circumstances that may occur during a student's clinical rotation; to provide the student with some experience, via role playing, in dealing with nonroutine events

Discussion

Students will be assigned a particular role from the situations outlined. Students are instructed to interject their own personalities into the role playing. Once a situation has been "played out" by the students, the instructor will lead a group discussion, covering the issue(s) presented in each situation.

Situation 1

Patient (Outpatient): Your physician has requested that you go to the laboratory to have your blood drawn for electrolytes and a CBC. You are terrified of needles because of your previous unfavorable experiences. You have been told that you have "terrible veins." Too much trauma causes you to faint.

Phlebotomist: Patient Robinson needs to have blood drawn for electrolytes and a CBC. Patient Robinson has informed you that his/her blood draw experiences in the past have been nightmarish. Patient Robinson has stated, "They always tell me that I have terrible veins."

Situation 2

Patient: You "hate" hospitals. You had a vacation to Hawaii scheduled, and instead of the Maui vacation you dreamed of, you landed up in this hospital! You are furious that you had to cancel your vacation plans! Out of everything you have had to endure since being admitted, the blood tests are the worst. This is absolutely the last time you will be "stuck" before talking to your physician. You have decided that the phlebotomist will get ONE chance only to obtain your blood!

Phlebotomist: This is your first day "on your own." Your first patient was easy. However, you were unable to secure a specimen from your second patient after 2 attempts. Furthermore, the last patient criticized your abilities. Your confidence has been shattered! You enter the room of Patient #3. You have requisitions for a glucose, prothrombin time, and type and crossmatch. You tried the patient's left arm and missed. (The patient had a good vein, but you missed it because you were so nervous.) The patient is becoming hostile.

Situation 3

Parents: Your only child (aged 1 year) is in the hospital. You are determined to spend every moment with the child and monitor the hospital's every move! You realize the child is ill, but you find it extremely difficult to watch the hospital staff come in and "stick" your child all day long. You plan to intervene the next time someone comes in. The child is tired, crying, and you think he has had enough for one day! (You will NOT leave the room!)

Phlebotomist: You walk into pediatrics. You have a requisition to draw a CBC on the 1-year-old child. The child's parents are in the room. You prefer to have parents leave the room when collecting blood specimens from their child.

Situation 4

Mary Surestick: You have been a phlebotomist for more than 10 years. You never got around to becoming certified. Now, in addition to everything else, you must help train phlebotomy students assigned to your facility for their phlebotomy rotations. The students almost always become certified shortly after completing their phlebotomy training. The hospital is exploring the possibility of revising the pay scale to financially reward certified phlebotomists. The students are slow, and it takes twice as long to do everything when they are involved. You have a requisition for a type and crossmatch and hemoglobin and hematocrit on Mr. Had Enuff. Mr. Enuff has brittle diabetes, and his glucose is drawn every 4 hours. You are very familiar with Mr. Enuff!

Phlebotomy Student: You have begun your clinical rotation at Hospital XYZ. You are assigned to work with Mary Surestick, a phlebotomist with 10 years of experience. You and Mary have a requisition for a type and crossmatch to be collected from Mr. Had Enuff. Upon locating Mr. Enuff, Mary Surestick identified him by glancing at the name card above his bed. Mary instructs you to collect the type and crossmatch on Mr. Enuff and says, "I've already identified the patient, just go ahead and draw him."

Situation 5

Phlebotomist: You are assigned to draw patients in the psychiatric department. When you walk into the intensive care part of the department, you see a friend of your younger sibling in leather restraints. You overhear 2 nurses talking at the nurse's station. They are discussing the patient who has had a drug overdose and is in leather restraints. When you return to the lab, the technologists are talking about the same patient and wondering how he lived after taking so much of the drug.

Sibling: When you went to school today, one of the "guys" you "hung around" with never showed up. Another person from your group of friends said he overdosed and was admitted to Hospital A. Hospital A is where your older sibling works as a phlebotomist. You want the "scoop" on your friend!

Situation 6

Phlebotomist: You are on your last patient for morning draw. The patient is an 85-year-old woman who seems really "out of it." Her bed is entirely soiled with fecal material. The odor in the room is unbearable. A chemistry profile and hemoglobin and hematocrit are ordered. What is the appropriate course of action?

Situation 7

Phlebotomist: You have recently begun working on the 3 PM to 11 PM shift at Hospital B. You were on the floor collecting 4 PM sugars and have just returned to the lab. You find 2 stat requisitions on the counter. One is a stat glucose from medical ICU and the second is a stat CBC from the medical/surgical floor. While you are examining the 2 stat requisitions, 2 more stats arrive. One is a request for a stat monospot from the emergency department, and the second is for a type and crossmatch from labor and delivery. No one else is available to assist in the collection of the 4 stats. How do you prioritize the stat requests? How would you deliver the blood specimens to the laboratory? How long should it take to collect all 4 specimens?

Situation 8

Patient: You were in an automobile accident. The ambulance took you to Hospital C, a teaching hospital. You do not like teaching hospitals because you prefer to have persons attend you who are already trained. You have decided not to let any students participate in your care.

Phlebotomist: You are in your last week of phlebotomy clinical rotation at Hospital C. Your instructors have indicated that your progress is remarkable. You have been offered a job at Hospital C and are scheduled to start next week! You are assigned to draw the patient described above.

Situation 9

Phlebotomist: You have a request for a stat CBC and BUN on the patient in Room 203, bed 1. When you enter the room, the patient's physician is with the patient. What should you do next? What takes priority: the stat request or the physician's conference with the patient?

Situation 10

Phlebotomist: You have just completed collecting blood specimens for cardiac enzymes and a prothrombin time. When you arrive at the nurse's station to report the blood was collected, the ward secretary informs you the physician has just ordered a stat CBC on the same patient.

What is the appropriate course of action?

Situation 11

Phlebotomist: Give an example of a patient who did not follow patient preparation guidelines. Create a scenario involving a patient who did not follow preparation guidelines. Indicate the role of the phlebotomist in the scenario you have created.

Situation 12

Below is an illustration of a ladder. The ladder represents your career as a health care worker. Each rung of the ladder represents your specific goals toward achieving success. Identify a goal for each rung on the ladder. Specify a date when you anticipate achieving each goal.

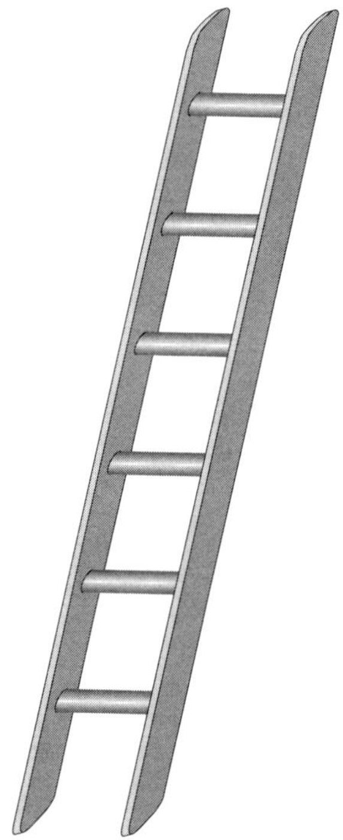

APPENDIX 1

Glossary

Afebrile: without fever

Agglutinin: antibody that causes aggregation (clumping) when reacted with a particular antigen

Anaerobic: without oxygen

Antecubital fossa: hollow or depressed area located in front of the elbow

Antimicrobial: the killing of microorganisms or inhibition of their growth

Asymptomatic: showing or causing no symptoms

Attenuated virus: the weakening of a virus prior to inoculation; may be accomplished through the use of heat, chemicals, growth in tissue culture, or desiccation

Bacteremia: the presence of bacteria in the bloodstream

Biohazard: substance, usually blood or body fluid, capable of transmitting disease

Cannula: apparatus used to access a vein for dialyzing and for blood drawing in patients with kidney disease

Carcinogenic: cancer producing

Causative agent: a body or substance responsible for a particular disease state

Caustic: burning or corrosive, destructive to living tissue

Collateral circulation: situation in which blood is provided to an area of the body by more than one blood vessel

Concentric: more than one circle, all of which have the same center

Continuum: line representing the sum total of all parts contributing to the line

Corrosive: destructive to the texture or substance of tissues

Dermis: the layer of skin beneath the epidermis; consists of a dense bed of vascular connective tissue

Diluent: an agent used to dilute (reduced in strength by intermixture)

Dilution: solution formed when an entity is mixed with a diluent

Distal: a position away from the trunk of the body

Emesis basin: kidney-shaped container used to collect vomit

Endemic: diseases that are present in a particular geographic area at all times

Endocarditis: inflammation of the membrane lining the chambers of the heart

False negative: a situation when a laboratory result is determined to be negative, when in fact it should be positive; may be biologic or the result of procedural error

False positive: a situation when a laboratory result is determined to be positive, when in fact it should be negative; may be biologic or the result of procedural error

Filtrate: a liquid that has passed through a filter

Fistula: structure formed by the surgical fusion of a vein and artery; used for dialysis in patients with kidney disease

Flora: may refer to bacteria normally found in a particular location, such as in the intestines and/or on the skin

Gangrene: death of tissue, often accompanied by loss of blood supply to the tissues and the resulting invasion of bacteria

Gauge: the bore size of a needle; the smaller the number used for gauge size, the larger the needle; the larger the number used for gauge size, the smaller the needle (eg, a 22-gauge needle is much smaller than a 16-gauge needle)

Geriatric: that branch of medicine that addresses the health and diseases of the elderly

Graduated cylinder: piece of lab equipment used to measure volume, mostly of fluids; shaped like a cylinder with a base on the bottom and a spout on top to enable pouring; marked with lines, or graduations, which correspond with the volume of fluid contained within the cylinder

Hematology: department of the clinical laboratory that is primarily responsible for the examination and quantization of blood cells

Hemoconcentration: decrease in the fluid portion of the blood; results in a higher hematocrit

Hg: chemical abbreviation for "mercury"

Hyperemia: an excess accumulation of blood in a localized area

Inoculation: the injection of a vaccine to protect the recipient from a particular disease

In vitro: term referring to within the laboratory

In vivo: term referring to within the living body

IV: abbreviation for intravenous

Lateral: away from the midline of the body (ie, toward the side of the body)

Medial: toward the center or midline of the body

Meniscus: the concave or convex upper surface of a body of liquid; when using a graduated cylinder, volumes are read from the bottom of the meniscus

Microbe: a minute living organism, including bacteria, fungi, and viruses

mm: abbreviation for millimeter

Morphologic: pertaining to structure or form

Needle disposal unit: container, usually manufactured of hard plastic, used to house discarded needles until the needles can be autoclaved or incinerated

Normal range: the numeric range of values for a particular test; most of the population will have values within the normal range

Nosocomial infection: an infection a patient acquires as the result of a hospital stay

Oncology: the branch of medicine that deals with tumor management and treatment

Osteochondritis: inflammation of both bone and cartilage

Palmar: the palm side of the hand

Pediatric: that branch of medicine that deals with children, their care, and the treatment of disease

Petechiae: small bruises the size of a pinpoint

Phalanx: any bone of the toe or finger

Plantar: the bottom of the foot (ie, the sole of the foot)

Polycythemia: abnormal increase in the red blood cell mass of the body

Primary atypical pneumonia: a type of pneumonia seen most often in children and young adults; caused by infection with *Mycoplasma pneumoniae*

Prophylaxis: the prevention of disease

QNS: abbreviation for quanitity not sufficient; the term may be used to reject a specimen if there is an insufficient amount to perform the analysis requested

Rouleaux: abnormal appearance of red blood cells, like a stack of coins

Sepsis: presence in the blood or other tissues of pathogenic microorganisms or their toxins

Septicemia: a systemic disease associated with the presence and persistence of pathogenic microorganisms or their toxins in the blood

Sphygmomanometer: blood pressure cuff

Stasis: reduction or stoppage of the flow of blood in a part of the body

Stethoscope: an instrument used to perform mediate auscultation

Subcutaneous: beneath the skin

Susceptibility: the state of being affected; in antimicrobial therapy, antibiotics to which the pathogen is susceptible are administered

Titer: (in reference to cold agglutinin titers) the highest dilution of a patient's serum that will cause the red blood cells to agglutinate (clump) in the test system

Toxoid: a bacterial exotoxin that is no longer toxic but can still elicit and combine with an antitoxin

Turgid: swollen and congested

APPENDIX 2

Blood Tests and Collection Requirements

CONTRIBUTED BY RAYMOND OLESINSKI, MHPE, MT(ASCP)PBT,SH, CLS (NCA)

TEST[1]	DEPARTMENT[2]	SPECIMEN REQUIRED[3]	COLLECTION TUBE[4]	SPECIAL HANDLING	CLINICAL RELEVANCE
Acetone	Chemistry	Serum	Red or SST	Chill specimen; do not use alcohol to cleanse puncture site	Diabetic coma
Acid Phosphatase	Chemistry	Serum	Red or SST	Chill specimen; avoid hemolysis	Prostate function
Acid Phosphatase, Prostatic	Chemistry	Serum	Red or SST	Chill specimen; avoid hemolysis	Prostatic cancer
Adrenocorticotropic Hormone (ACTH)	RIA[5]	Plasma (EDTA)	Lavender	Chill specimen	Adrenal function
Alanine Aminotransferase (ALAT, SGPT)	Chemistry	Serum	Red or SST		Hepatic function
Albumin	Chemistry	Serum	Red or SST		Hepatic & renal function
Alcohol	Chemistry	Serum	Red or SST	Do not use alcohol to cleanse puncture site	Alcohol intoxication
Aldolase	RIA	Serum	Red or SST	Separate and freeze serum if testing is delayed	Muscle disease
Alkaline Phosphatase	Chemistry	Serum	Red or SST		Hepatic function, bone metabolism
Ammonia	Chemistry	Plasma (Heparin)	Green	Chill specimen	Hepatic failure & Reye's syndrome
Ampicillin	TDM[6]	Serum	Red or SST	Indicate if peak, trough or random collection	Antibiotic monitoring
Amylase	Chemistry	Serum	Red or SST		Pancreatic function
Antibody Screen	Blood Bank	Whole blood (ACD), Serum, and Cells	Yellow (ACD) or Red		Screen for presence of abnormal antibodies
Antinuclear Antibody (ANA)	Immunology	Serum	Red or SST		Systemic lupus erythematosus
Antistreptolysin O (ASO) Titer	Immunology	Serum	Red or SST		Streptococcus infection
Antithrombin III	Coagulation	Plasma (Sodium citrate)	Light Blue	Separate plasma and freeze if testing is delayed	Screen for thrombotic tendencies
Aspartate Aminotransferase (ASAT, SGOT)	Chemistry	Serum	Red or SST		Hepatic & cardiac function
Bilirubin	Chemistry	Serum	Red or SST	Shield specimen from light; avoid hemolysis	Hepatic function
Blood Culture	Microbiology	Whole blood (SPS)	Yellow (SPS) or suitable culture medium bottles	Cleanse tube or bottle stoppers with iodine prior to filling to avoid contamination; collect before specimen tubes	Bacteremia

TEST[1]	DEPARTMENT[2]	SPECIMEN REQUIRED[3]	COLLECTION TUBE[4]	SPECIAL HANDLING	CLINICAL RELEVANCE
Blood Urea Nitrogen (BUN)	Chemistry	Serum	Red or SST		Renal function
Calcium	Chemistry	Serum	Red or SST		Parathyroid function
Carcinoembryonic Antigen (CEA)	RIA	Serum or plasma (EDTA)	Red, SST or Lavender		Monitor progress of carcinoma
Carotene (Vitamin A)	Chemistry	Serum	Red or SST	Shield specimen from light; avoid hemolysis	Screen for steatorrhea
Catecholamines	Chemistry	Plasma (Heparin)	Green	Collect specimen from indwelling needle after patient has been supine for 30 minutes; chill specimen	Adrenal function
Cholesterol, High-Density Lipoprotein (HDL)	RIA	Serum	Red or SST		Cardiac risk monitoring
Cholesterol, Total	Chemistry	Serum	Red or SST		Cardiac risk monitoring
Cold Agglutinins	Blood bank, Immunology	Serum	Red	Clot & separate serum from cells; do not use serum separator tube; maintain specimen at 37°C until serum separation; avoid hemolysis	Atypical pneumonia
Complement, Total	Immunology	Serum	Red or SST	Separate & freeze serum if testing is delayed	Immune system function
Complete Blood Count (Usually includes WBC, RBC, HGB, HCT, MCV, MCH, MCHC, platelet count, and possibly MPV, RDW and 3-part differential)	Hematology	Whole blood (EDTA)	Lavender	Refrigerate if testing is delayed; avoid hemolysis	Anemia, infection
Coombs', Direct	Blood bank	Serum & cells	Red	Do not collect in serum separator tubes	RBC absorption of antibodies
Copper	Chemistry	Serum	Royal Blue		Hypercupremia, Wilson's disease
Cortisol	RIA	Serum or plasma (EDTA or heparin)	Red, SST, Lavender or Green		Adrenal function
C-Reactive Protein (CRP)	Immunology	Serum	Red or SST		Inflammatory disease
Creatine Kinase (CK) (Creatine Phosphokinase [CPK])	Chemistry	Serum	Red or SST		Cardiac function
Creatine Kinase (CK) Isoenzymes (Creatine Phosphokinase [CPK] Isoenzymes)	Chemistry	Serum	Red or SST	Separate serum and freeze if testing is delayed	Myocardial infarction
Creatinine	Chemistry	Serum	Red or SST		Renal function
Cytomegalovirus (CMV) Antibody	Immunology	Serum	Red or SST	Fasting specimen	CMV infection

TEST[1]	DEPARTMENT[2]	SPECIMEN REQUIRED[3]	COLLECTION TUBE[4]	SPECIAL HANDLING	CLINICAL RELEVANCE
Digoxin	TDM	Serum	Red or SST		Cardiac medication monitoring
Dilantin® (Phenytoin)	TDM	Serum	Red or SST		Seizure medication monitoring
Drug Screening	Chemistry	Serum	Red or SST		Screen for substance abuse/overdose
Electrolyte Profile (Na, K, Cl, CO_2)	Chemistry	Serum or Plasma (Lithium or ammonium heparin)	Red, SST, or Green	Avoid sodium heparin anticoagulant; avoid hemolysis	Fluid balance; cardiac, renal, & pulmonary function
Electrophoresis, Protein	Chemistry	Serum	Red or SST		Hepatic and renal function
Eosinophil Count	Hematology	Whole blood (EDTA)	Lavender		Allergy, parasitic infection
Epstein-Barr Virus (EBV)	Immunology	Serum	Red or SST		Screen for EBV infection
Erythrocyte Sedimentation Rate (ESR)	Hematology	Whole blood (EDTA or potassium oxalate)	Lavender or Black		Inflammation
Erythromycin	TDM	Serum	Red or SST	Indicate if peak, trough or random collection	Antibiotic monitoring
Estriol	RIA	Serum or plasma (EDTA or heparin)	Red, SST, Lavender or Green		Female hormone monitoring
Estrogen (Estradiol)	RIA	Serum or plasma (EDTA)	Red, SST or Lavender		Female hormone monitoring
Factor Assay(s) (Coagulation Factors II, V, VII, VIII, IX, X, XI, XII and/or XIII)	Coagulation	Plasma (Sodium citrate)	Light Blue	Separate plasma and freeze if testing is delayed	Factor deficiencies
Febrile Agglutinins	Immunology	Serum	Red or SST		Bacterial & parasitic infection
Fibrin Degradation Products (FDP, FSP)	Coagulation	Serum	See Special Handling	Collected in Thrombo-Wellcotest tube or equivalent	Disseminated intravascular coagulation (DIC)
Fibrinogen	Coagulation	Plasma (Sodium citrate)	Light Blue	Blue-stoppered tube must be completely filled; chill specimen	Disseminated intravascular coagulation (DIC), Factor I deficiency
Fluorescent Treponemal Antibody (FTA)	Immunology	Serum	Red or SST		Screen for syphilis
Folate	RIA	Serum or whole blood (EDTA)	Lavender	Separate serum or plasma from cells and freeze immediately	Anemia
Follicle-Stimulating Hormone (FSH)	RIA	Serum	Red or SST		Female hormone monitoring
Fungus Antibodies, Complement Fixation	Immunology	Serum	Red or SST		Screen for fungal infections
Gamma-Glutamyl Transpeptidase (GGTP)	Chemistry	Serum	Red or SST		Hepatic function

TEST[1]	DEPARTMENT[2]	SPECIMEN REQUIRED[3]	COLLECTION TUBE[4]	SPECIAL HANDLING	CLINICAL RELEVANCE
Gastrin, Serum	RIA	Serum	Red or SST	Patient should fast 12 hours before collection; chill specimen	Gastric malignancy
Gentamicin	TDM	Serum	Red or SST	Indicate if peak, trough or random collection	Antibiotic monitoring
Glucose	Chemistry	Serum or plasma (Potassium oxalate/ sodium fluoride, heparin, EDTA)	Red, SST, Gray, Green, Lavender	Collect in gray-stoppered tube if testing will be delayed. Indicate if sample is fasting, postprandial or random.	Diabetes screening, diagnosis & monitoring
Glucose-6-Phosphate Dehydrogenase (G-6-PD)	Hematology	Whole blood (EDTA)	Lavender		Genetic enzyme deficiency
Group and Rh Typing	Blood bank	Serum & cells	Red	Do not collect in serum separator tube	ABO & Rh determination
Haptoglobin	Immunology	Serum	Red or SST		Hemolytic anemia
Hematocrit	Hematology	Whole blood (EDTA)	Lavender		Anemia
Hemoglobin	Hematology	Whole blood (EDTA)	Lavender		Anemia
Hemoglobin A_{1C}	RIA	Whole blood (EDTA)	Lavender		Diabetes monitoring
Hemoglobin Electrophoresis	Hematology	Whole blood (EDTA)	Lavender		Abnormal hemoglobin determination
Hemoglobin, Plasma	Hematology	Plasma (Heparin)	Green	Collect specimen gently with syringe; remove needle and dispense into open collection tube; stopper and invert gently; avoid hemolysis	Hemolytic anemia
Hepatitis A Antibody	RIA	Serum	Red or SST		Screen for exposure to hepatitis A
Hepatitis B Surface Antibody	RIA	Serum	Red or SST		Screen for exposure to hepatitis B
Hepatitis B Surface Antigen (HBsAg)	RIA	Serum	Red or SST		Screen for hepatitis B carrier state
Hepatitis C Antibody	RIA	Serum	Red or SST		Screen for exposure to hepatitis C
Hepatitis D Antibody	RIA	Serum	Red or SST		Screen for exposure to hepatitis D
Herpes Simplex Antibody	Immunology	Serum	Red or SST		Screen for herpes simplex infection
Heterophile Agglutination	Immunology	Serum	Red or SST		Infectious mononucleosis
HIV Antibody Screen	Immunology	Serum	Red or SST		Screen for HIV seroconversion
HIV Antibody Confirmation	Immunology	Serum	Red or SST		Confirmation of HIV seroconversion
Human Chorionic Gonadotropin HCG()	RIA	Serum or plasma (EDTA)	Red, SST or Lavender		Pregnancy testing

TEST[1]	DEPARTMENT[2]	SPECIMEN REQUIRED[3]	COLLECTION TUBE[4]	SPECIAL HANDLING	CLINICAL RELEVANCE
Immunoglobulins (IgG, IgA, IgM and/or IgD)	Immunology	Serum	Red or SST		Myeloma
Infectious Mononucleosis Screen	Immunology	Serum	Red or SST		Infectious mononucleosis screen
Insulin	RIA	Serum	Red or SST		Glucose metabolism
Iron & Total Iron-Binding Capacity	Chemistry	Serum	Red or SST		Iron deficiency anemia
Kanamycin	TDM	Serum	Red or SST	Indicate if peak, trough or random collection	Antibiotic monitoring
Ketones	Chemistry	Plasma (Potassium oxalate/sodium fluoride)	Gray	Chill specimen	Diabetic acidosis
Lactate (Lactic Acid)	Chemistry	Plasma (Potassium oxalate/sodium fluoride)	Gray	Do not have patient clench fist during collection; chill specimen	Gastric malignancy
Lactate Dehydrogenase (LDH)	Chemistry	Serum	Red or SST	Avoid hemolysis	Hepatic & cardiac function
Lactate Dehydrogenase (LDH) Isoenzymes	Chemistry	Serum	Red or SST	Avoid hemolysis	Hepatic & cardiac function
LE Prep	Hematology	Plasma (Heparin)	Green		Systemic lupus erythematosus
Lead	Chemistry	Plasma (Heparin)	Brown		Lead intoxication screen
Leucine Aminopeptidase (LAP)	Chemistry	Serum	Red or SST		Hepatic function
Lipase	Chemistry	Serum	Red or SST		Pancreatic function
Lithium	Chemistry	Serum	Red or SST		Antidepressant drug monitoring
Luteinizing Hormone (LH)	RIA	Serum or plasma (EDTA)	Red, SST or Lavender		Female hormone monitorin
Magnesium	Chemistry	Serum	Red or SST		Fluid balance
Malaria, Blood Smear	Hematology	Plasma (EDTA)	Lavender		Malaria
Osmolality	Chemistry	Serum	Red or SST		Respiratory & fluid balance
Osmotic Fragility	Hematology	Plasma (Heparin)	Green		Hemolytic anemia
Parathyroid Hormone (PTH)	RIA	Serum	Red or SST	Chill specimen	Parathyroid function
Partial Thromboplastin Time, Activated (APTT)	Coagulation	Plasma (Sodium citrate)	Light Blue	Evacuated tube must be completely filled	Coagulopathy, heparin therapy
Penicillin	TDM	Serum	Red or SST	Indicate if peak, trough or random collection	Antibiotic monitoring
pH	Chemistry	Plasma (Heparin)	Green	Chill specimen	Respiratory & fluid balance
Phosphate (Phosphorus)	Chemistry	Serum	Red or SST		Parathyroid function

TEST[1]	DEPARTMENT[2]	SPECIMEN REQUIRED[3]	COLLECTION TUBE[4]	SPECIAL HANDLING	CLINICAL RELEVANCE
Platelet Count	Hematology	Whole blood (EDTA)	Lavender		Coagulopathy
pO_2, pCO_2	Chemistry	Arterial whole blood (Heparin)	Use heparinized syringe	Chill specimen; seal specimen to avoid contact with room air	Respiratory function
Prothrombin Time (PT)	Coagulation	Plasma (Sodium citrate)	Light Blue	Evacuated tube must be completely filled	Coagulopathy, Coumadin® therapy
Protoporphyrin, Erythrocyte	Chemistry	Plasma (Heparin or EDTA)	Brown, Green or Lavender	Shield specimen from light	Congenital erythropoietic protoporphyria
Rapid Plasma Reagin (RPR)	Immunology	Serum	Red or SST		Screen for syphilis
Renin	RIA	Plasma (EDTA)	Lavender	Chill specimen	Hypertension
Reticulocyte Count	Hematology	Whole blood (EDTA)	Lavender		Anemia
Rheumatoid Arthritis (RA) Screening	Immunology	Serum	RED or SST		Screen for rheumatoid arthritis
RhoGAM Workup	Immunohematology	Whole blood (ACD), Serum, and Cells	Yellow (ACD) or Red		Determine eligibility for RhoGAM injection
Rubella Screening	Immunology	Serum	Red or SST		Screen for rubella
Sickle Cell Screening	Hematology	Whole blood (EDTA)	Lavender		Screen for sickle hemoglobin
Strep Screen	Immunology	Serum	Red or SST		Strep infection screening
T_3, T_4 & T_7	RIA	Serum	Red or SST		Thyroid function
Theophylline	TDM	Serum	Red or SST		Asthma medication monitoring
Thrombin Time	Hematology	Plasma (Sodium citrate)	Light Blue	Evacuated tube must be completely filled	Coagulopathy
Thyroid-Stimulating Hormone (TSH)	RIA	Serum	Red or SST		Thyroid function
T-Lymphocytes, Helper & Suppressor (T4 & T8)	Immunology	Both whole blood (EDTA) and plasma (Heparin) required	Lavender & Green	Prepare fresh blood smears from EDTA specimen	Immune function
Tobramycin	RIA	Serum	Red or SST	Indicate if peak, trough or random collection	Antibiotic monitoring
Total Protein	Chemistry	Serum	Red or SST		Hepatic & renal function
Toxoplasma Antibody Screening	Immunology	Serum	Red or SST		Screen for Toxoplasma infection
Triglycerides	Chemistry	Serum	Red or SST	Patient should fast 8–12 hours prior to collection	Cardiac risk monitoring, diabetes mellitus

TEST[1]	DEPARTMENT[2]	SPECIMEN REQUIRED[3]	COLLECTION TUBE[4]	SPECIAL HANDLING	CLINICAL RELEVANCE
Type & Crossmatch (T & C)	Blood bank	Serum & cells	Red	Do not collect in serum separator tubes; avoid hemolysis	ABO & Rh typing & compatibility testing
Type & Screen	Blood bank	Serum & cells	Red	Do not collect in serum separator tubes; avoid hemolysis	ABO & Rh typing & antibody screening
Uric Acid	Chemistry	Serum	Red or SST		Gout, renal function
Vancomycin	TDM	Serum	Red or SST	Indicate if peak, trough or random collection	Antibiotic monitoring
Varicella Zoster Immune Status	Immunology	Serum	Red or SST		Determine antibody levels to varicella zoster virus (chickenpox)
VDRL (Venereal Disease Research Labs)	Immunology	Serum	Red or SST		Screen for syphilis
Vitamin B_{12}	RIA	Serum or whole blood (EDTA)	Red, SST or Lavender	Shield specimen from light	Anemia
White Blood Cell Count (WBC)	Hematology	Whole blood (EDTA)	Lavender		Infection, leukocyte disorders
White Blood Cell Differential (WBC Diff)	Hematology	Whole blood (EDTA)	Lavender		Infection, leukocyte disorders
Xylose Absorption (D-Xylose)	Chemistry	Plasma (Potassium oxalate/sodium fluoride)	Gray	Requires patient ingestion of xylose 1–2 hours prior to testing	Intestinal malabsorption

Notes

1. This list is provided as a guideline for student use. It is not a complete list of currently available laboratory procedures, but provides details on some of the more commonly ordered tests. The menu of procedures available will vary from laboratory to laboratory.
2. The usual department that has responsibility for performing a test is given. Department designations and responsibility may vary from lab to lab.
3. The information in parentheses indicates the anticoagulant and/or additive of the evacuated tube used for specimen collection. Specimen requirements may vary by methodology and from lab to lab.
4. Colors of collection tubes correspond to those of the VACUTAINER tubes (without HEMOGARD closure) manufactured by Becton Dickinson. SST corresponds to collection tubes containing serum separator gels. Stopper colors and additives may be different for other manufacturers' tubes.
5. Radioimmunoassay
6. Therapeutic drug monitoring

Bibliography

Henry JB. *Clinical Diagnosis and Management by Laboratory Methods.* 17th ed. Philadelphia, Pa: WB Saunders; 1984.

Midwest Laboratory Reference Manual. Chicago, Ill: MetPath; 1992.

Pendergraph GE. *Handbook of Phlebotomy.* 3rd ed. Philadelphia, Pa: Lea & Febiger; 1992.

Slockbower JM, Bruck E, Calam RR, et al. *Procedures for the Collection of Diagnostic Blood Specimens by Venipuncture.* 3rd ed. Villanova, Pa: National Committee for Clinical Laboratory Standards; 1984.

APPENDIX 3

Profile Test Groups

Sometimes physicians will order tests in groups called profiles. Listed below are examples of profiles commonly ordered. Specific tests included in a profile vary with each facility.

Profile Name	Tests Included	Sample Required
Chemistry profile	Glucose, blood urea nitrogen (BUN), creatinine, sodium, potassium, chloride, alanine aminotransferase (ALAT), aspartate aminotransferase (ASAT), lactate dehydrogenase (LDH), bilirubin, alkaline phosphatase, amylase	15 mL red or 15 mL red SST
Complete blood count (CBC)	Hemoglobin, hematocrit, WBC count, RBC, mean corpuscular hemoglobin (MCH), mean corpuscular hemoglobin concentration (MCHC), mean corpuscular volume (MCV), differential	Lavender top
Coagulation profile	Prothrombin time (PT), activated partial thrombo-plastin time (APTT), platelet count, bleeding time	1 blue top, 1 lavender top, bleeding time
Prenatal profile	ABO group and Rh type, antibody screen, rapid plasma reagin (RPR), rubella, CBC	2 red tops, 1 lavender top
Immunology profile	Antistreptolysin-O (ASO) titer, C-reactive protein (CRP), rheumatoid arthritis (RA) screen and titer, complement levels, immunoglobulin levels	3 red tops
Cardiac profile	Total cholesterol high-density lipoprotein (HDL), low-density lipoprotein (LDL), triglycerides, cardiac enzymes, creatine kinase (CK), aspartate aminotransferase (ASAT), and lactate dehydrogenase (LDH)	2 red tops

APPENDIX 4

Bibliography

Blood Specimen Collection by Skin Puncture in Infants. Rutherford, NJ: Becton Dickinson; 1980.

Brown B. *Hematology: Principles and Procedures*. 3rd ed. Philadelphia, Pa: Lea and Febiger; 1980.

Bruck E, van Assendelft OW, Jacoby H, Schulman J. H3-A2. *Procedures for the Collection of Diagnostic Blood Specimens by Skin Puncture*. 2nd ed. NCCLS; 1992.

Henry JB. *Clinical Diagnosis and Management by Laboratory Methods*. 17th ed. Philadelphia, Pa: WB Saunders Co; 1984.

Enforcement Procedures for Occupational Exposure to Hepatitis B Virus and Human Immunodeficiency Virus. Washington, DC: Occupational Safety and Health Administration, Office of Health Compliance Assistance; 1990.

Finegold SM, Martin WJ. *Diagnostic Microbiology*. St. Louis, Mo: CV Mosby Company; 1982.

Garner JS, Favero MS. *Guideline for Handwashing and Hospital Environmental Control*. Washington, DC: US Department of Health and Human Services; 1985.

Garner JS, Simmons BP. CDC guidelines for isolation precautions in hospitals. *Guidelines for Prevention and Control of Nosocomial Infections*. Washington, DC: US Department of Health and Human Services; 1983.

Garza D, Becan-McBride K. *Phlebotomy Handbook*. 3rd ed. East Norwalk, Conn: Appleton and Lange; 1993.

Gloss SB, Plunkett PF. *Arterial Blood Gas Sampling* [slide/videotape]. Denver, Colo: Multi-media Publishing; 1984.

Holland P, ed. *Standards for Blood Banks and Transfusion Services*. Arlington, Va: American Association of Blood Banks; 1989:B1.263.

Klosinski D, Miller C, Narlock V. *Blood Collection: The Routine Venipuncture* [videotape and monograph]. Chicago, Ill: ASCP Press; 1989.

Klosinski D. *Blood Collection: The Difficult Draw* [videotape and monograph]. Chicago, Ill: ASCP Press; 1993.

Kotter ML. *A Programmed Guide to Medical Terminology*. Dubuque, Iowa: Kendall/Hunt Publishing Co; 1981.

Luebbert PP. *Laboratory Safety and Infection Control* [videotape and monograph]. Chicago, Ill: ASCP Press; 1990.

Luebbert PP. *OSHA's Bloodborne Pathogens Standard: Compliance in the Clinical Laboratory* [videotape and monograph]. Chicago, Ill: ASCP Press; 1992.

Microcollection Inservice Material [videotape, wall chart, pocket reference card]. Rutherford, NJ: Becton Dickinson Vacutainer Systems; November 1991.

Musgrave KA, Triplett DA, Daly CH, Schlossberg L, Bausback AG. The art and science of the bleeding time test. *ASCP Check Sample*. Chicago, Ill: American Society of Clinical Pathologists.

Pendergraph GE. *Handbook of Phlebotomy*. 3rd ed. Philadelphia, Pa: Lea and Febiger; 1992.

Phelan S. *Blood Collection: Special Procedures* [videotape and monograph]. Chicago, Ill: ASCP Press; 1991.

Phelan S. *Blood Collection: The Pediatric Patient* [videotape and monograph]. Chicago, Ill: ASCP Press; 1990.

Phelan S. *Phlebotomy Techniques Curriculum Guide.* Chicago, Ill: ASCP Press; 1993.

Recommendations for prevention of HIV transmission in health care settings. *MMWR*. 1987;36:2S.

Slockbower JM, Belgeri K, Bruck E, et al. H4-A2. *Procedures for the Collection of Diagnostic Blood Specimens by Venipuncture*. 2nd ed. NCCLS; 1986.

Slockbower JM, Blumenfeld TA. *Collection and Handling of Laboratory Specimens*. Philadelphia, Pa: JB Lippincott Co; 1983.

Stansfield WD. *Serology and Immunology: A Clinical Approach*. New York, NY: Macmillan Publishing Co; 1981.

Update: universal precautions for prevention of transmission of human immunodeficiency virus, hepatitis B virus, and other bloodborne pathogens in health care settings. *MMWR*. 1988;37:24.

Williams WW. CDC guideline for infection control in hospital personnel. In: *Guidelines for Prevention and Control of Nosocomial Infections*. Washington, DC: US Department of Health and Human Services; 1983.